THE EXERCISE CURE

A Doctor's
ALL-NATURAL, NO-PILL
Prescription for
Better Health & Longer Life

Jordan D. Metzl, MD,

with Andrew Heffernan, CSCS

RODALE.

"The first wealth is health."
—RALPH WALDO EMERSON
(1802–1882)

Around the world every day, there are hundreds of millions
of people working to make their lives healthier in both mind and body.
Each person has their own issues, their own struggles.
They all share a universal goal, however, to better themselves.

I dedicate this book, and the information inside,
to those seeking self-improvement. May the knowledge in these pages
help springboard you to a healthier version of yourself.

Contents

PART 1

The Miracle Drug You Need to Take

I magine yourself at your next doctor's appointment. The doc walks into the office, sits down across from you, looks you in the eye, and says, "Good news, I can help you. I'm writing you a prescription and I want you to follow it to the letter."

"What is it?" you ask.

"It's a miracle drug," he replies.

You chuckle. "Sorry, doctor, but I really don't believe in miracles."

He nods as if expecting you to say that, then says: "You will."

"I doubt it," you reply.

"Well, what if I told you that this drug treats *everything*? And what if I told you that this drug helps prevent almost every illness you *might* get, including certain types of cancer? And that it's 100 percent effective, and it works for every person around the world, rich or poor, young or old, with no side effects?"

"That's crazy," you say. "There's no such thing."

The doctor only smiles . . . and begins telling you all about this mythical, magical miracle drug. . . .

+ + +

First of all, he says, it's the weight-loss drug millions have been waiting for. It's very simple: If you use this drug, you will lose weight in a totally healthy way. Imagine, he says, the implications for the obesity crisis. And for those who have weight-related health issues, the drug gives immediate benefits. In the endocrine system, for example, research has shown that this miracle drug can reduce the progression of type 2 diabetes by 58 percent. For some patients who stay on this drug long-term and increase their dosage, type 2 diabetes can be reversed.

For the cardiovascular system, the drug prevents heart disease. It immediately helps address hypertension (high blood pressure) and hypercholesterolemia (high cholesterol) and greatly reduces your chance of suffering a heart attack or a stroke. And if you've already been diagnosed with heart disease or related problems? This drug helps improve your condition.

How about everyday health problems? This drug boosts your immune system against common maladies like the cold and flu, reducing the intensity and duration, or preventing them outright.

In your brain, the drug can block the progression of dementia and Alzheimer's by up to 50 percent. The drug has also been shown to help you keep your mental faculties longer in life, and it will keep your brain working better and longer compared to those who refuse to take it.

If we stay in your head and look at psychological factors, the drug also works wonders. It's been shown to reduce symptoms of depression by 30 percent, and closer to 50 percent in higher doses ("That's the beauty of this drug," says the doctor. "It's very hard to O.D."). It's also incredibly

THE ONE THING YOU CAN DO TODAY TO LIVE LONGER

Exercise.

Yes, there's that word again. But as you'll read, more and more research has emerged showing that exercise lengthens life.

Consider just this one piece of research: A 2012 study in the journal *PLOS Medicine* showed that 2.5 hours of moderate exercise per week (that's half an hour of brisk walking a day for 5 days) increased life expectancy by 3.5 years.

Those in the study who upped their exercise intensity increased life expectancy by 4.2 years.

Understand that this wasn't a small group of college students measured over a few weeks. This review looked at data of more than 600,000 people.

That's one thing you can do today to extend your life.

Exercise.

effective against anxiety disorders. The drug attacks low energy and boosts self-esteem. It lets you work at a higher level for a longer time. It can help you quit any addiction and is especially effective with smoking and drinking. This medicine improves sleep quality and can cure sleep disorders like insomnia and apnea.

Also, and this is a big one, we know that chronic low-level inflammation in the body plays a key role in causing some of the worst diseases we have: heart disease, arthritis, Alzheimer's disease, Parkinson's disease, asthma, irritable bowel syndrome, and more. Our miracle drug, when used regularly, helps tame inflammation in the body, thus helping prevent all of these nasty outcomes.

The drug also helps make your body indestructible (or, at least, a lot less likely to break down). For the skeleton, it makes bones stronger and muscles less likely to be injured. In older people, this drug aids in mobility and prevents falls. Postmenopausal women who took this drug four times a week had a 47 percent lower risk for hip fracture. And folks in one study took this drug and saw their knee arthritis pain reduced by almost half.

That's part of the miracle in this miracle drug: The more you take it, the more active you become. This drug can make you better at your favorite sport. It helps you jump higher, run faster, and improve your flexibility and coordination.

Last but not least: This drug even helps prevent certain types of cancer

THE SIMPLE SELF-TEST YOU NEED TO TAKE RIGHT NOW

Brazilian researchers figured this one out, and I think every doctor should give this test to every patient. If anything, it will open everyone's eyes to the importance of regular exercise. Here's what to do:

Sit on the floor. Indian-style is fine. Now: Stand. Do so without worrying about speed, and do so with the absolute minimum help you need (whether it comes from using your hands, another person, a wall, or furniture).

That's it. That's the test. What does it prove?

The researchers tested 2,000 men and women ages 51 to 80. Those who could stand up without using their hands or getting other help lived longer than those who couldn't. A *lot* longer. Those who got up on their knees and needed help from a table or wall or another person to stand were *six times* more likely to die prematurely than the nonhelp group. Why?

This very simple test reveals *everything* about your current strength, flexibility, and coordination. In this research group, those who could rise using just one hand, or with no help at all, were in the top 25 percent for musculoskeletal fitness.

It's so simple: The higher your fitness level, the longer you'll live.

The people in this study were older, but I'll bet there are a lot of younger people out there who would have a tough time standing up without any help.

Take it to heart, folks, and take this test. If you have trouble with it, I hope it inspires you to start a regular exercise program (lots of ideas in this book!). Even if you do something as simple as adding pushups, planks, and lunges to your daily activity, you'll see a huge difference when you retest yourself only a few weeks later.

Try it. Your life may depend on it!

and can help you fight back if you ever get a diagnosis.

"But I lied," says the doctor. "There are side effects."

"See? I knew it," you say. "Let me guess: Deadly rash and uncontrollable drooling."

The doctor laughs. "Not quite. There are two side effects: Every single person who takes this medicine decreases their risk of premature death, and every single person who takes this medicine raises their quality of life."

The doctor leans back and lets all of this sink in.

"Okay, Doc," you say. "If everything you say is true, then every doctor in the world who didn't prescribe this medicine to every patient that came in would be committing medical malpractice."

Your doctor looks at you and smiles. "One hundred percent correct. So let's talk about how you're going to fill your prescription. . . . "

By now you've guessed it. The miracle medicine that works across every disease state is called exercise.

And everything I just told you is true. Science has shown again and again, across all manner of diseases, maladies, and health risks, that exercise can prevent, improve, or outright cure your symptoms. As a sports medicine physician and an avid athlete myself, I've written this book to teach you how to maximize your dose of the world's most effective medicine.

I Prescribe This Medicine Every Day—To Myself

What I'm about to tell you would be considered "anecdotal evidence" in research circles. Not long ago, those who touted the benefits of exercise were thought of as outliers or "fringe." But now that science has caught up, I can tell you one thing for certain: I see the incredible medical benefits of exercise every single day when I look in the mirror. I love exercising. It keeps me happy. It keeps me healthy. (I hardly ever get so much as a head cold.) It also helps me help others and put forth a positive example to my patients. I walk the walk (or run the run, as it were). I've completed 11 Ironman triathlons and 30 marathons, and I teach hard-core Iron Strength fitness classes on the weekends. Without regular exercise, I don't know what I'd do.

I got a taste of that while I was in medical school.

During my first year, I was playing soccer and blew out my knee (when you hear the expression "A first-year med student could diagnose that," that was me, writhing on the grass screaming my diagnosis: "I tore my ACL!"). For the first time in my life, I was sidelined and dealing with serious doubts about whether or not I'd ever be able to be a competitive athlete again.

Folks, those were dark days for me. I was depressed and scared. I'd lost the one thing that kept me happy and healthy. Both my mental and physical health had been compromised because I was told to "stay off it," and because I really didn't know how the knee would respond to rehab after surgery.

I realized that I performed better as a student when I exercised—and I couldn't exercise. Instead, I had to find ways to stay active even with an injured knee. To this day, I use many of these same techniques with my patients. Throughout my medical career, exercise enables me to focus and perform my best. And I learn even more as I go. About 5 years ago, I walked into the strength class of my friend Dejuanna Richardson and discovered the benefits of kinetic chain strengthening as a way to decrease joint impact. Instead of achy knees, I learned to make my knees feel better by building the muscles around them. Now I teach my own strength classes.

So obviously, things turned out okay. But I'm a perfect example of how lack of exercise changes everything for you.

I also see the benefits of exercise when I race and when people show up for my classes. Yes these folks are sweating and pushing hard, but they're also enjoying it. And when they're done, they're smiling ear to ear.

And finally, I see the benefits of exercise in my practice with my patients. When someone comes in with a sports injury, they're in the same boat I was in: scared and depressed. But they don't have to be, and I let them know it up front. I never prescribe "total rest." After all,

they have other body parts they can work while the injured part heals. (I'll talk more about this in the special section later in this chapter.) Plus, humans are built for movement. Movement makes us happy. Lying around watching the world pass by makes us sad—and all you have to do is compare depression rates between people who move and people who don't to know that that's true. So once my patients understand that they can keep exercising other body parts while the injured parts heal . . . again, the ear-to-ear smile.

But what about you? I assume you've come to this book—the way patients come to my office—because you don't feel as good as you should.

Good news: I can help you. This book can help you. How do I know? Besides the hundreds of tips and plans and bits of science and pieces of advice inside, this book, at its core, is a feel-good book. Or maybe a feel-*better* book.

You see, millions of people in our society suffer from a ridiculous number of health problems—some major, some minor that could become major—because they lack basic fitness. Meanwhile, my goal in life is to keep myself and as many people as possible moving in a positive direction. So I'm glad you're here!

I suspect you know exactly what I'm talking about because you picked up this book. You read the cover and thought, *Hmm, what's this all about?* But that is just a surface thought. Deeper down, where there's just you and the truth, you're looking for an

Lack of Exercise Is Expensive

Want to save money? Exercise.

Based on current estimates, the United States spends more than $2.6 trillion—17 percent of the gross national product—on health care. That's $8,300 per person. And somehow we rank 28th in the world for life expectancy.

Regular exercise is the key to a longer, healthier, and *less expensive* life.

answer. Your life and health aren't what they could be. You know it. You want to change it. You're not sure how. And here you hold a book called *The Exercise Cure.*

I'll say it again: This book will help you. But first, you need to be inspired. Emotions drive all our decisions, for better or worse, and if I can elicit that positive emotional response, if I can convince you simply to *move*, then a big part of my job is already done.

So right here, right now, I want to inspire you. I want you to read this book and feel deep down that positive change is simple. That feeling better every day is a real promise. That all you have to do is stand up and move to guarantee yourself a healthier and longer life.

It's true. It's real. You hold in your hands the secret to improving, preventing, or curing many health problems. How? One word:

Exercise.

That's a loaded word. For most people, they hear it and have an immediate response: On the outside, they nod like they understand, because, hey, everyone knows they should exercise. But on the inside? They bristle, or groan, or cringe. Because, hey, everyone knows they should exercise. Inspiring people to exercise is one tough job, believe me.

Every day you hear what I call the "magazine cover" promises of exercise: *Strip away fat! Sculpt your abs! Look better naked!* If those promises inspire you to exercise regularly, awesome. That makes me happy. And hey,

those magazines sell millions of copies, so the message works for some.

I want to dig a little deeper, however. Here's the line I wish magazine editors would splash across every single cover they publish: *Exercise is medicine!*

No less than the American College of Sports Medicine has made that its motto. Thousands of doctors have spent decades researching exercise and treating millions of people for these "self-inflicted" health problems caused by lack of fitness. The result is undisputed: Exercise is honest, inexpensive, all-natural medicine. It's also the easiest, cheapest, and fastest way to a happy life. When formerly sedentary people start moving regularly, miraculous things happen—just as miraculous as any treatment or procedure or drug I've ever seen or prescribed in my medical career.

It's all so simple, and I'll keep saying it: I want you to maximize your dose of the world's most effective medicine. This book will show you how. And by doing that, I hope to inspire you to improve every facet of your health and life.

Let's take that first step together, right now.

How the "Miracle Drug" Works

When I say, "Exercise is medicine," one of the most common questions I get is, "What do you mean?" I'll show you.

A SCARY COMPARISON

A lot is written about the overall health (or lack of it) of our society. A lot is also written about one of the biggest problems facing the United States: rising federal and personal debt levels. Don't worry, this isn't a political rant. It's a simple illustration of what you're doing to yourself if you ignore fitness and choose lying on a sofa instead of working up a sweat.

Anything you do that is bad for your health is the equivalent of racking up huge amounts of debt.

It's simple math: If you carry a lot of debt, you're kicking your financial problems down the road. You'll pay for it tomorrow, or the next day. But make no mistake, whether you pay it off by sacrificing something valuable or find yourself choking on debt payments months or years from now, *you will pay*. And you'll possibly destroy your credit score and financial future. After all, you can't "retire rich" with a credit card balance.

The math is just as simple for unhealthy activities.

• **You don't exercise.** You're racking up a huge health debt that you will indeed pay for—possibly with your life—in the future. And make no mistake, *you will pay*.

• **You eat too much.** Excess calories will be stored as fat, but this is not like putting money in a savings account. It's like jacking up your credit card balance. The more fat you store, the more "health debt" you have to carry, and the bigger the bill down the road.

• **You drink too much.** Hitting the booze too hard is both a short-term and long-term health debt. Sure, you have a sensational night. But tomorrow you pay with your hangover. And if you drink too much over a period of years, the health debt comes due in the form of everything from liver and pancreatic problems to weakened blood vessels. And if you *really* mess up? A car accident or DUI.

You get the idea—and it applies to *any* unhealthy activity. Now, do the math in the opposite direction: If you exercise, eat right, and live a reasonably healthy lifestyle otherwise, you're making an investment in your future. You're banking good health outcomes for later. How? Well, let's say you're fit and physically stronger than the average person because you exercise. If you experience some kind of health emergency that requires medical treatment, possible surgery, and significant recovery time, your physical fitness will make that entire process easier, and your recovery shorter. Why? A fit body bounces back faster than an unfit body.

Again, the math is really simple. Make the smart choices.

In 2003, K.C. Maurer, a patient and friend of mine who is a CFO in Manhattan, was spending Memorial Day weekend at her summer home at the Jersey Shore. While hanging drapes, she felt a sudden, stabbing pain in her chest, followed by intense nausea. In the emergency room, she found out she'd suffered a heart attack. She was 41 at the time.

"I was so surprised," she recalls. "I told the doctor, 'You must have mixed up the blood work.'"

Like the rest of her family, K.C. was heavy: 330 pounds at 5 foot 6 inches tall. But she was hardly inactive. Like a lot of New Yorkers, she walked miles every day, hustling from one social or work obligation to the next, and figured her activity level and fitness would save her from serious health risks. At her doctor's urging, K.C. hired a nutritionist and began getting more serious about her workouts.

Despite losing nearly 40 pounds and improving her diet, K.C. suffered two more heart attacks the following year. "It was frustrating," she told me. She was doing everything right—why was this happening?

K.C. was undeterred. Instead of giving up on physical activity, she doubled down on it, setting her sights on completing the 2005 New York Marathon. Pouring rain and a strict cutoff time forced her to abandon the race at mile 18, but, man, she still ran 18 miles! Very few people can do that. She was inspired. She resolved to return the following year and complete the course.

Three days before the '06 marathon, K.C. found herself in the hospital again—this time for a kidney stone. But a CAT scan showed a rare, hard-to-detect tumor on an adrenal gland that her doctors later determined had been the cause of her multiple heart attacks. Suddenly, on top of everything else, she was staring down the barrel of a possible cancer diagnosis.

K.C. surprised everyone, even herself, with her response to the diagnosis: "My first question for the doctor wasn't 'Will I live?'" she says. "It was 'Will I get to do the race?' The prospect of not racing was worse than the tumor itself." She would later recognize it as the moment she became an athlete.

A few days later, K.C. completed the New York Marathon. Her nutritionist, her cardiologist, and four out-of-town college friends greeted her at the finish line. High-fives and hugs all around. She'd done it: In the 3 years since her first heart attack, she'd completely revamped her eating habits, become a dedicated exerciser, and fierce competitor—and dropped 110 pounds in the process.

Since then, K.C. has completed 3 more marathons and 29 half-marathons. Along the way, she fought back against obesity, diabetes, and a cancer scare—not to mention heart disease—and emerged victorious. These days, K.C. regularly speaks to groups of women about heart health. "I tell them that even if you're starting off at 330 pounds and multiple

THE EXER-CYCLE

Exercise isn't just medicine. Regular vigorous activity can set a cycle in motion that builds and builds in positive ways as you go around and around. Start with "Do Your Workout Today!" and follow the arrows to see how your life will change for the better—all from working up a simple sweat.

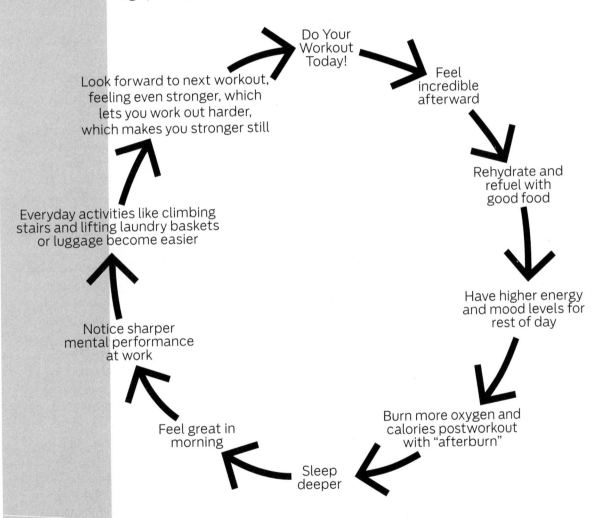

Do Your Workout Today!

Feel incredible afterward

Rehydrate and refuel with good food

Have higher energy and mood levels for rest of day

Burn more oxygen and calories postworkout with "afterburn"

Sleep deeper

Feel great in morning

Notice sharper mental performance at work

Everyday activities like climbing stairs and lifting laundry baskets or luggage become easier

Look forward to next workout, feeling even stronger, which lets you work out harder, which makes you stronger still heart attacks in your 40s, you can still transform yourself.

"Regular exercise makes me feel as if I can conquer any challenge I'm confronted with, physical, mental, spiritual," she says. "It helps me solve problems, gives me perspective, and keeps stress at bay."

Could she have done it without exercise? It's possible to lose weight through diet without exercise, yes. But her fitness goals didn't just require exercise, they *inspired* it. It transformed her physically. Frequent, vigorous movement improved her blood pressure, lowered her blood sugar, thinned her blood, strengthened her heart, and muscled up her immune system. Exercise-induced hormones lifted her mood, helped her focus on her work and on accomplishing the next goal. Her entire body got stronger. She lost fat. Her bones thickened. And, just as important, her daily exercise habit, and the ever-present goal of finishing the next race, reminded her that she was strong and capable, even in the face of some very tough health challenges.

"I used to be motivated by fear," she concludes. "Fear of dying, being sick, and being a burden to family and friends. Now I'm motivated by a desire to be worthy of my two god-daughters, Ava and Adele. I want them to know that setbacks and failure are possible—and sometimes necessary—in order to achieve the best life possible. There is a big world out there, and I want to squeeze as much joy out of life as I can. That's not going to happen if I just sit on the couch."

Let me introduce you to another extraordinary woman. Just over 20 years ago, New York City–based art teacher Elaine Breiger was diagnosed with breast cancer. While undergoing treatment, which is hard enough by itself, she decided on a whim, and with no training to speak of, to enter the New York Marathon. She completed the race (in 6 hours and 16 minutes), loved it, and soon after began running seriously. Since then she has completed dozens of marathons, improving her time steadily. These days, her cancer is in full remission and she sometimes walks away with a first-place medal in her age group: women, age 80 to 84.

Yes, you read that right. In addition to running up to 50 miles a week, this octogenarian strength trains twice a week, teaches full-time, and paints.

Exercise didn't cure Elaine's cancer. But it certainly made her stronger—and inspired—during her fight. And though I didn't know her in her youth, I imagine she was bright and energetic long before she took up endurance racing. Anyone dealing with aging, chronic disease, or simply the day-to-day pressures of life would do well to follow her example. Asked what keeps her going, she'll tell you, "I figure it's either move or rust in peace."

IS EXERCISE BETTER THAN "REAL" MEDICINE?

I'm up-front about the therapeutic properties of exercise. Science and my own experience bear this out. But I don't want you to misunderstand: Just because you exercise regularly, "real" medicine (in the form of procedures, pills, or any other method used to treat illness and injury) should never be ignored or avoided if you have a health problem.

I practice and strongly believe in Western medicine. I've been trained in the most current disease treatments the world has ever known. Western medicine is literally lifesaving for millions every year: If you have end-stage kidney disease, we can replace the kidney; if you have an arthritic hip, we can replace the hip; or if your coronary artery is clogged, angioplasty can change your prognosis overnight. Even something as simple as an antibiotic can save your life.

That said, I get this question all the time: "Is exercise better than 'real' medicine?" The answer is, "It depends." If you're having a heart attack as we speak, obviously you need an ER, not a gym. But after you're treated and have recovered enough to be cleared by your doctor, exercise is *crucial* medicine both to help you fully recover and to prevent another heart attack.

Another example: A type 2 diabetic may need medication to manage his or her condition. But regular exercise could help improve the condition to the point where meds may no longer be necessary. Exercise can also get you off cholesterol, blood pressure, and other common drugs, if your doctor sees enough improvement to warrant it.

My point is, a medical problem sometimes requires several methods of treatment. But exercise, in some instances, can gradually reduce the number of methods necessary until the only treatment you need is exercise itself.

In short: I'd like for you to use the information in this book *in addition to* Western medicine, not instead of it.

Ice Cream? Beer? Nope, Here's *What's Really Killing You*

My years in med school and, later, encountering shining examples of smart exercise habits in my professional practice, have taught me that the common denominator among many health problems out there, major and minor, is *low fitness.*

It really is that simple, and that important. More than once, when a patient has come to see me for a problem, I've have the urge to write "EXERCISE" on my prescription pad—above and beyond everything else—because exercise truly would be the best medicine for what ailed him or her at the time. Now, in this book, I can literally give you specific exercise prescriptions for different problems or to improve a general lack of fitness.

Many talking heads would have you believe that obesity is destroying our health. That's true, to a point. Being overweight hurts you in many ways. But a lot of good research has shown that *low fitness* is a bigger predictor of premature death, no matter how much you weigh. I'm not the only one who believes this.

A couple of years ago, Dr. Steven Blair from the University of South Carolina's Arnold School for Public Health quantified the effects of various health risks on the likelihood of dying for a group of 50,000 men and women. Blair calculated how much less likely it was for a person to die if he or she eliminated certain risk factors: if a smoker kicked the habit, for example, or if an obese person lost the extra baggage.

Low fitness stood out by far as the single strongest predictor of death—more powerful even than obesity, diabetes, high cholesterol, high blood pressure, and smoking. With the exception of high blood pressure, which ran a close second, compared to the risks associated with being unfit, the other factors were small potatoes. It wasn't even close. In fact, the research shows that if you're highly fit when in your eighties, you're less likely to die than if you're unfit when in your sixties.

Think about that for a moment, folks.

That means if you're a middle-aged, obese smoker with high blood pressure, high cholesterol, and diabetes, *the single best thing you can do to improve your health is exercise.* Not simply as a way to lose weight (you will). Not simply so you can "feel better" (you will), raise your self-esteem (you will), or fit into your high school jeans (you will if you decide that's what you want). But to save your life.

Add to that the obvious fact that exercise will directly lower the risks associated with many other health problems, and you have a pretty compelling case for working out on a regular basis.

In some cases, exercise is such effective medicine that it works better than *actual* medicine. In 1999,

WHY I RECOMMEND YOU EXERCISE 7 DAYS A WEEK

I'm a big proponent of exercising every day. Not many people are willing to do this. Some will say they don't have the time. More accurately, they won't make time. Some say they want to rest their bodies, let themselves recover from the previous day's workout. Well, human bodies are designed for everyday use. Our ancestors, from the caves to the farm fields, got their butts out the door early and sweated all day, every day. We can certainly find 30 minutes to an hour to break a sweat, no? The key is to avoid overuse. How do you do this?

Change it up. If you weight train primarily, go for a bike ride or take a yoga class. If you jog, lift some weights. Do something for fun. You'll see several terrific yet challenging options in this list. Some other suggestions: Find a pool. Play Ultimate Frisbee. Or maybe just get out for a brisk walk with your dog.

Some other helpful hints:

- Exercise with friends and make it social.

- Set a fitness goal or make a friendly wager.

- Experiment with new sports, new equipment, or even a new playlist on your iPod.

I look at daily exercise as a healthy addiction. We have so many obesity-related health issues that are not treated until after they happen. Hypertension and diabetes are preventable with daily exercise. Exercise *is* medicine, preventive medicine, and it needs to be a daily ritual just like brushing your teeth.

You don't want to overdo it, of course. Listen to your body.

My point is, a body that is used *sensibly* every day grows accustomed to being used and won't be as prone to injury.

for example, James A. Blumenthal, PhD, professor of psychiatry and behavioral sciences at Duke University, compared three treatments for depression. One group took an antidepressant; another did moderate, regular exercise; and a third group did both.

Guess what? All three groups saw relief from their symptoms. Case closed? Not so fast: Six months later, over a third of the two *medicated* groups had relapsed into depression. The exercise-only group, by contrast, *relapsed at a rate of only 8 percent.*

The findings suggest that exercise not only combats depression better than medication—it works better than exercise and medication *combined.* If you're depressed, in other words, exercise should be your number one line of defense. There's a reason that exercise has become known as "nature's antidepressant."

And unlike many mood-altering medications, exercise won't blunt your libido or cause weight gain. Quite the opposite for both.

In another study, researchers compared a surgical intervention with an exercise program for preventing heart attacks in people who'd formerly had heart problems. One group had stents implanted to clear

THE MYSTERIOUS MAGIC OF EXERCISE

We all know that exercise builds muscle and endurance. And if you've read this far, you're probably starting to understand how it can build your immune system, boost your mood, and protect you from chronic disease. But what about that old high school coach chestnut, *character*? Can regular exercise build that as well?

New research suggests that, in a sense, it can: In a 2006 study published in the *British Journal of Health Psychology,* researchers found that sedentary people placed on an exercise program voluntarily began smoking less, drinking fewer alcoholic and caffeinated drinks, and eating healthier. More mysteriously, they also did more household chores, used their credit cards less often, and kept up more diligently with study and work obligations. Everything in their lives that required self-discipline, in other words, became easier—almost by magic.

"Regular exercise builds self-regulatory resources," explains Dr. Todd Heatherton, a professor of psychology and brain sciences at Dartmouth College and an expert in habitual behavior and addiction. And this ability to self-regulate, or exert willpower, say researchers, may be the most significant key to success in virtually any environment: It's what allows you to stick to a task when others give up and to overcome obstacles that at first seem insurmountable.

And somehow, regular exercise makes all that come more naturally.

arterial blockage. Another group rode stationary bikes 20 minutes a day and did hour-long aerobics-style fitness classes once a week.

Again, both interventions worked, but the exercisers fared better: Stents prevented heart problems over the next year in 70 percent of the people who received them. The exercise program, however, staved off heart problems over 12 months *an amazing 88 percent of the time.*

Strong numbers—especially when you consider that the exercisers did not have to pay for their treatment or stay in a hospital or undergo surgery. They also derived many other head-to-toe benefits from their workout programs, which the patients who received stents, obviously, did not. The only side effects brought on by exercise were things like improved mood, better focus, healthier body composition, and other bennies that the best pills in the world couldn't hope to provide. I'd venture to guess that the exercisers even enjoyed their treatment—far more, anyway—than those who received surgery.

Any health care practitioner worth his or her stethoscope will tell you that it's always cheaper and easier to avoid illness than it is to treat it. Unfortunately, our current health care system is much more concerned with treating and managing disease than it is with prevention—which may be part of why we spend so much on health care ($300 billion

annually on prescription medications alone), and yet have worse health outcomes than many countries that spend less.

Your Fitness: The Ignored "Vital Sign"

Go to a checkup and your health care provider will almost certainly check your weight and blood pressure, listen to your heart, and ask you about your smoking habits. But it's much more uncommon for them to inquire about or assess your fitness level—despite the research showing that low fitness is such a huge contributor to chronic illness.

Most doctors will tell you that there just isn't time, and it's not a priority, especially when a patient has come to them with a specific and pressing health concern. They're right; the system isn't set up for fitness measurement. And of course there's the practical issue of having people do situp drills and timed 50-yard dashes down hospital corridors to test their fitness levels (though I imagine some of my patients might really enjoy that). I *really* like the sit-and-stand test I mentioned earlier in the chapter. That one is simple enough to perform in an exam room.

But the fact is that we don't give prevention its due. I do my best to emphasize it with my patients and to impart smart exercise habits to the people who attend my weekly exercise classes. But I'm just one doctor. Given how important prevention is for both the individual and the society at large, we should be offering more incentives for people to stay healthy, just as we offer them incentives for having kids, getting married, and getting an education. We should find ways to subsidize wellness in the same way that insurance companies subsidize major surgeries and expensive medications (okay, I'll get off my soapbox; I couldn't resist).

Now: As a doctor, I'll tell you that I always want to be of help to whoever walks into my office. I want to be able to offer patients clear directives that will make their lives easier and more comfortable. I imagine many other doctors feel the same way. So it's not the easiest thing—or the most natural thing—for me to look a patient in the eye and say, "This one's on you, buddy."

But maybe we should be doing just that.

In 2009, the American College of Sports Medicine, a worldwide network of health professionals dedicated to promoting physical fitness through scientific research and education, launched a global initiative called *Exercise Is Medicine*. Their vision is to:

WORK OUT, GET RICH?

3 Ways That Health Makes Wealth
It turns out that exercise is medicine for your career, as well. White-collar warriors often believe that time away from the office is money lost. But research is showing that all work and no play not only makes Jack a dull boy, but a poorer one as well. Here's what regular exercise can do for your bottom line:

• **It impresses the higher-ups.** You might think time-crunched upper management types wouldn't have bandwidth for exercise, but these days very few fat cats are actually fat. In a 2005 survey, researchers found that 75 percent of top executives believed that physical fitness was "critical to career success," and that being overweight was a "serious impediment" to advancement. Want that promotion? Get thee to the gym.

• **It gives you a leg up.** Taking care of yourself gives you an edge over less-fit coworkers who don't. A 2010 study indicated that slender women outearn their overweight colleagues by a significant margin, and that men of moderate weight earn more than thinner men *and* heavier men. Talk about sweat equity.

• **It improves your attitude.** Endorphins are real: A 2008 study found that 45 to 60 minutes of a midday group exercise class improved the mood, performance, and concentration of white-collar workers. Workers only got these benefits on days when they exercised, however. So though you may be tempted to ditch your workout on days when there's an important meeting or project scheduled, you probably should make it even more of a priority.

1. Make exercise a standard part of a global disease prevention and treatment paradigm and

2. Consider physical activity and fitness level as a vital sign in every patient visit—just as blood pressure, heart rate, and pupil response would be during an annual physical. And also to counsel and refer patients in accordance with their physical activity and health needs, thus leading to overall improvement in the public's health and long-term reduction in health care cost.

I think they're on to something.

Now, I'm not ready to hang up my stethoscope and tell you that exercise is the cure for everything that ails you. Real maladies require real medicine in the form of diagnosis, treatment, medication, and other interventions like surgery. That's why most entries in the system-by-system malady section you're about to read has a section called "When to Call a Doctor" for guidance on professional advice and what you can expect when you get it. What I hope I've made clear in this introduction, though, is that if you have a health problem, major or minor—or, equally, if you're seeking to stave *off* health issues—the number one solution is often simply to *move*.

This book will show you how to do just that. In the section that follows, I go through a list of common ailments and take you through what the latest science tells us about the exercise prescription for preventing, or helping to treat, each one.

That's just the beginning. No matter what your fitness level, the workout sections give you an endless combination of exercises, plans, and intensity levels so you'll never be bored and never plateau. Just getting up off the sofa? No problem. Training for a marathon? I can make you stronger. My workouts can be tailored to any fitness need or goal. Finally, I give you a full chapter on how to fuel your exercise with the right food, the right amounts, and at the right time. Exercise requires fuel, after all, and smart eating will help you perform better and reach your ultimate goal: health and happiness.

My hope is that this book will help motivate and guide you in the best ways to get and stay active—whether you're dealing with extra weight or other health issues right now, or whether you're trying to prevent illness and get into the shape of your life while you're at it. Either way, you've taken the best first step. I'll be right there to keep you motivated and inspired. And always, always, always, remember to have fun. One thing I've learned after all these years as a doctor and an athlete: Exercise is that much sweeter when you do it with a smile.

SPECIAL SECTION
What If You Get Hurt Exercising?

Use "dynamic rest" to keep moving and heal at the same time!

Reality: Exercise can cause injury. Even the most diligent injury-prevention techniques aren't fool-proof. Every active person has aches and pains and things worse than that. And I hate to say it, but simple bad luck stalks us all. When pain strikes, there's one piece of advice I need to give you.

If you get hurt . . . KEEP MOVING!

What does that mean?

An injury is not a vacation from fitness or exercise. You must continue to work out even if you need to rest another body part so it can heal. There are specific reasons for this, reasons that I've learned firsthand in my experience as a doctor and an athlete. There are also smart ways you can keep exercising without aggravating the body part that's hurt.

But first, the WHY:

Years ago, as I mentioned, I blew out my knee in med school—a torn ACL that I eventually had to have surgery to repair. It kept me sidelined for a long time. And I'd never been sidelined before. I believe that the feel-good neurotransmitters secreted during exercise, like serotonin and dopamine, are very much drug-like, and exercise is one of our healthiest drugs. So when it's taken away it can be clinically depressing for people. That's *exactly* how I felt when I hurt my knee and couldn't exercise.

That's why I believe, as a doctor and an athlete, that when you're hurt, total rest and "staying off it" is not just unwise, it's medically unhealthy.

Think about it: What happens when you can't do any physical activity?

You become bored. Your mind drifts into negativity. The research showing a positive mind-body connection through exercise is undeniable; "nature's antidepressant," remember? I've noticed myself that young athletes in school have lower academic performance when they're injured. More time on your hands isn't always a good thing.

You miss your regular dose of feel-good neurotransmitters. Besides the pain of the injury, you simply don't feel as good as you normally do.

Your body atrophies. And not just your skeletal muscles. The heart is a muscle, and like any other muscle, if you take 4 weeks off to rest something, that muscle atrophies and your cardiovascular condition deteriorates. You'll have a lot of work to get back to where you were (thus the old adage "It's easier to stay in shape than to get in shape.").

You endure depression. I've felt it. I had surgery to fix the ACL, and aside from the painfulness of the experience that I hope I never repeat, the 6 months to a year of rehab and only gradual ability to get back to the sports I loved was mental torture.

It was also enlightening.

You need to keep moving to fight all those negatives I just described. You'll keep some of your conditioning. You'll get your dose of neurotransmitters. You'll feel better. You'll be more positive. And you'll learn that no injury is the end of the world.

So . . . how do you exercise while injured?

Do what I call *dynamic rest* That means two things.

One, rest and rehab—lay off the injured body part and do what you need to do to get it back to health. That could mean basics like ice and compression or something specific prescribed by a doctor like targeted physical therapy or exercises.

And two, be dynamic, stay in motion as all this rest and rehab goes on. That's the trick. Here's how:

• **Find an activity that doesn't interfere with the injury you have.** If you sprain your ankle, for example, do something that doesn't load your ankle. Hit the pool. Hit the upper-body weight training hard. Bad knee? Same concept. Whatever your injury, find its opposite counterpart and work it. Bad shoulder or elbow? Run and do lower-body plyometrics. And here's a big one: Bad back? Simply move. Walk. Shuffle if you have to. But resting a bad back only deconditions the muscles and makes it weaker. No matter what body part hurts, find something that doesn't aggravate it, but DO NOT do "complete rest."

• **Go hard.** Whatever your alternate activity is, up the intensity. This will get your heart pounding and your lungs heaving and keep your cardiovascular system in shape. Heck, it might even improve it. It'll also release those giddy neurotransmitters and you'll be the happiest hurt person on Earth.

As you can see, injuries can hurt you, but they don't have to halt you. Exercise is one of the most important things we have for lifelong health and happiness. It's real preventive medicine. It doesn't just make you feel good. It keeps you from feeling bad. Don't let anyone or anything take that away from you.

PART 2

What Seems to Be the Problem?

Here's your go-to guide to a host of common health problems—some dangerous, some debilitating, but all of them a hindrance to a healthy and happy life. Each entry in this section is packed with information: key symptoms, a breakdown of how and why the problem occurs, as well as who has the highest risk. I'll also give you my specific exercise prescription for each case—sometimes as simple as getting off the couch, sometimes as detailed as an entire workout (these are in addition to the workouts I offer in Part 3). Understand, however, that no matter how good you think you are at self-diagnosis (and perhaps denial), there are definitely times when you need to see a professional for your problem. I cover that, too. The "When to Call a Doctor" boxes will give you the facts on making that all-important appointment and what to expect. Good luck, and here's to health and happiness!

CHAPTER 1

Brain and Psychological Problems

Neurologists used to believe that movement affected only the primitive areas of the brain, and that the more evolved areas—such the prefrontal cortex—were reserved for "higher" functioning: social interaction, planning, and emotional intelligence.

Turns out that the areas of the brain affected by movement are interlaced throughout the whole organ. Said one neurologist I know, "There's hardly a cell in your brain that isn't profoundly affected by movement." That means that you can directly affect your emotional centers by taking a run. You can literally light up your brain's decision-making circuitry with a trip to the weight room.

More and more, it's clear that exercise is a remarkably potent "way in" that helps us avoid, improve, and sometimes even solve psychological problems—from stress to sleep problems, from fatigue to addiction. Exercise and movement of all kinds grow and organize the brain in a very powerful and direct way that we're only starting to understand. So get moving—and start feeling better.

THE PROBLEM:
Addiction

THE SYMPTOMS: You're drawn to some type of mood-altering behavior or substance, and you keep giving in to it, despite negative consequences. Symptoms include preoccupation with your drug or behavior of choice, a lack of control over it, and continued use despite adverse consequences. Another big sign: denial that a problem exists. If it feels good now, feels awful later, and you can't stop yourself from doing it, chances are it's an addiction.

WHAT'S GOING ON: Addictions come in many forms, some of which can cause physiological dependency, others of which are, more accurately, intense forms of compulsive behavior.

In the case of *physiological dependency*, the body begins to rely on the substance to function properly and needs more and more of it to achieve the original, euphoric feeling (this is called *tolerance*). When the substance is removed, withdrawal symptoms occur, and the person needs to go through a period of detoxification in order to relearn how to function without it. Common withdrawal symptoms include acute cravings for your drug of choice, headaches, cold sweats, anxiety, tremors, irritability, nausea, and hallucinations. Smoking, drugs, alcohol, and some medications can lead to this type of dependency.

Other behaviors, including gambling, playing video games, watching and obsessing over sports, and using pornography can be addictive to varying degrees, as can some types of behavior that are usually considered beneficial—including calorie-restricted dieting, sex, and even exercise. And a newer addiction: social media. Some people really do need their "Facebook fix."

Depending on the person and the substance, an addiction can take hold overnight or over many years.

Why do addictions happen? People typically have a genetic predisposition to addictive behavior—if your parents are addictive types, you are more likely to be as well. But addiction has an environmental component, too, as you can't become addicted to something you've never experienced (which is why the first one's always free).

At some point, the addictive substance or behavior gets hard-wired to a biochemical process in the brain, which creates an illusion of euphoria, relaxation, and happiness when you experience your drug or behavior of choice, and an increasing desire for and preoccupation with the drug. The behaviors around obtaining the drug, and hiding your use of it, may further add to the allure of the addictive substance.

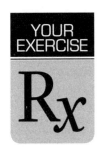

YOUR EXERCISE

Rx

Exercise can help combat virtually any addiction (except exercise addiction, naturally). Says one 2011 study, published in *Current Neuropharmacology*, "Exercise leads to an increase in the synthesis and release of dopamine, stimulates neuroplasticity and promotes feelings of well-being. Moreover, exercise and drugs of abuse activate overlapping neural systems." Researchers have theorized that this might explain why regular exercise helps to prevent addiction from taking hold—and can play a role in curing it as well.

In many studies, exercise has been shown to have a pacifying effect on addictive behavior. It blunts the urge to take drugs, gamble, and smoke, for example. A review of studies published in 2012 looked at the effect of exercise in people who were trying to quit smoking. Several of the studies reviewed showed "significantly" higher abstinence rates for the groups that exercised versus those that didn't. In this study, two groups of rats were exposed to amphetamines: one group of normal rats, another group that had a fully ingrained exercise habit. The exercising rats showed no preference for amphetamines, whereas the nonexercisers couldn't get enough of them.

Overall, this may explain why, statistically, exercisers are much less

(continued)

When to Call a Doctor

This can be problematic. Most addicts will never call a doctor or even ask for help with their problem. They believe they can handle it. Or they don't want to face it. Even with family interventions, an addict won't pursue real change until he or she is ready. And "ready" can be a long way off and include some horrifying consequences for the addict and those close to him or her. If you know an addict, seek professional guidance *for* them (and for yourself on how to handle the problem), and try to help as best you can. If you're an addict, deep down you probably know it. Even if you can't imagine a life without your addiction of choice, that better life is out there. There is no shame in admitting you need help—and the professional help out there is very real and very effective if you commit to it.

likely than inactive people to become addicts.

Another study, however, conducted by the Beckman Institute for Advanced Science and Technology at the University of Illinois in Urbana-Champaign in 2012, offers a different and perhaps somewhat qualified perspective of the value of exercise in overcoming addiction.

Two groups of mice—one habituated to exercise, the other not—were exposed, and became addicted to, liquid cocaine. The formerly sedentary mice were then *also* habituated to exercise. When the cocaine was taken away from both groups, the mice that had only taken up exercise *after* exposure to cocaine were able to break

their addiction much more easily than those who had the exercise habit in place *before* exposure. In some cases, the poor previously exercise-addicted mice continued to crave cocaine for the rest of their lives.

So does this mean that we shouldn't begin an exercise program unless and until we have an addiction to overcome? Or that exercising regularly will make you *more* susceptible to addiction?

It's hard to say: Mice aren't people, after all, and it was just one experiment. The big-picture lesson, say the researchers, may be that exercise primes the brain to learn, and adopt, new behaviors—regardless of whether those behaviors are self-

WHEN EXERCISE IS THE ADDICTION

Yes, it's possible. You can be addicted to exercise (the very definition of "too much of a good thing"). It stands to reason: Exercise can induce physiological pleasure responses the same way a drug can. Motor activity stimulates the release of dopamine, a naturally occurring narcotic in the brain that is also stimulated by many addictive substances and behaviors, including cocaine and methamphetamine. Natural endorphins, enkephalins, and endocannabinoids (opium- and marijuana-like substances also manufactured in the brain) also get in on the act.

There are signals for exercise addiction in both mind and body. In the mind: Does it dominate your life? Will you be seriously derailed for the day if you don't

exercise? In the body: chronic overuse injuries. All these are signs that you're exercising in unhealthy ways and should talk to your doctor about it.

In my own case, I'm probably a borderline exercise addict. I need it every day and I recommend it every day for my patients. I watch myself carefully. I'll ask myself, "If I'm going to give up a workout, why? Am I going to miss a dinner I should go to, or an important meeting, or a special occasion?" I'm pretty good about this, but not perfect. And that's the overall point of this entire section: Recognizing your own addictive tendencies—stepping back and seeing your own behavior—is a huge part of recognizing a potential problem.

destructive or beneficial. (This seems to be true at any age, by the way).

For you and me, that may mean that if you're trying to adopt or break a habit—be it eating less sugar, smoking fewer cigarettes, or shaking an Internet jones—you might want to begin or make a change in your exercise program *at the same time:* Start jogging or cycling or switch from rock climbing to martial arts, for example. The fresh neurons that your new or unfamiliar exercise program stimulates may make it easier to adopt the new behavior you're trying to master.

To recap:

- Exercise helps prevent addiction from taking hold.

- Exercise can help overcome addictive behaviors once they have taken hold.

- If struggling to overcome an addiction (or adopt a new behavior in general), you may benefit from making a change in your exercise program at the same time.

THE PROBLEM:
Anxiety

THE SYMPTOMS: You're worried, concerned, and fearful, generally about some threatening event in the future over which you feel you have little control. You may feel nauseated, shaky, experience blurred or tunnel vision, a racing heart, fatigue, the frequent need to go to the bathroom, panic attacks, and difficulty concentrating.

WHAT'S GOING ON: Anxiety can arise as a normal response to an upcoming frightening or stressful situation. In some circumstances, the response may actually provide a helpful cue that prompts you to confront a nagging or difficult problem, or helps you avoid a dangerous situation. Studies have shown that people with anxiety are, in fact, less likely to die in accidents.

Performance anxiety, stage fright, or fear preceding a test or evaluation are all common forms of anxiety. A certain amount of arousal is necessary for high performance, of course—too much, however, can hinder performance.

But, like depression and other mood disturbances, anxiety can also come up for no clear reason, attached to no obvious external threat or event, and ultimately become debilitating. Obsessive-compulsive disorder, phobias, and social anxiety are all clinical forms of anxiety and should be treated with help from a health care provider.

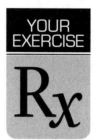

Exercise can be a powerful tool in preventing anxiety in the first place: People who exercise consistently are 25 percent less likely to develop anxiety than those who don't. In cases of mild anxiety, exercise can be extremely helpful, easing symptoms in just a few minutes, and though it can't cure chronic anxiety, it can help diminish its symptoms.

• **TRY YOGA.** Anxiety is often accompanied by a response from the sympathetic nervous system— the "fight or flight" response that prepares you for challenging physical activity. If you're chronically anxious, this system is probably working overtime, keeping your mind racing and your body keyed up, even when you're trying as hard as you can to calm down.

A 2011 review of research published in the *British Journal of Sports Medicine* found promising evidence that yoga may help relieve the symptoms of some types of mild anxiety—probably because the slow, languid movements and focus on deep breaths help stimulate a parasympathetic, calming response from the autonomic nervous system. Two or three classes a week of yoga can be very beneficial in this regard. And once you get the hang of it, you can try a little yoga breathing or a few *asanas* (yoga poses) whenever you feel symptoms of anxiety start to come up.

- **GO FOR THE GOLD.** Another study, published in 2005 in *Behavior Research and Therapy,* found that regular aerobic exercise also reduced anxiety and "anxiety sensitivity," or the fear of the sensation of anxiety itself, and that a higher intensity of this type of exercise worked better than a lower intensity. So if you're anxious, hit up the gold standard of exercise as described in Part 3—and skew your aerobic workouts a little tougher.

When to Call a Doctor

Intense and ongoing anxiety can take a toll on your life, cutting into productivity and leisure time. If anxiety is starting to become chronic and unmanageable, see a doctor. If left untreated, anxiety can become a debilitating disorder. Exercise is terrific treatment for a mild anxiety disorder, but the more serious variants need the help of a trained mental health professional.

THE PROBLEM:
Attention-Deficit Hyperactivity Disorder (ADHD)

THE SYMPTOMS: In children, an inability to concentrate, as well as difficulty following directions, sticking to tasks, and accomplishing household chores and schoolwork. Children with ADHD are easily bored and distracted, and often have difficulty sitting still and controlling their impulses.

In adults, ADHD often manifests in difficulty with time management, organization, goal setting, and emotional control—all of which can interfere with employment and relationships. Depression, low self-esteem, substance abuse, and addiction disproportionately affect adults with ADHD.

WHAT'S GOING ON: ADHD can be a very frustrating condition, both for the children and adults it affects and for those around them. Its exact causes are unknown, though heredity, chemical imbalances, and traumatic head injury may contribute to the condition. Women who eat poorly, smoke, or abuse drugs or alcohol during pregnancy are also more likely to give birth to children with ADHD.

ADHD is a behavioral condition and has no physical symptoms—though a doctor may take x-rays or a blood test to rule out any underlying physical conditions. Other psychological conditions, such as anxiety and depression, can cause similar symptoms, so doctors or specialists will take a thorough medical and personal history to verify the diagnosis.

ADHD does not come on in adulthood but is a lifelong condition. If, as an adult, you suspect you may have ADHD, a specialist will focus questions on your behavior, development, and relationships starting at childhood to determine the root cause of your condition.

Treatments for ADHD include prescription medications and various types of psychosocial interventions, including psychotherapy, behavioral modifications, special education, and social skills training. Left untreated, children with ADHD are at greater risk for teen pregnancy, car accidents, and drug and alcohol use. They are also more likely to have learning disabilities.

Since its causes aren't fully understood, ADHD can't be cured or prevented. But behavioral interventions, and drugs, if necessary, can go a long way in helping to regulate impulsive behavior and to help an affected child grow up to be productive and successful. Another helpful treatment: exercise.

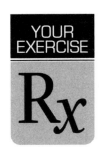

YOUR EXERCISE

Recent research suggests that exercise can be very effective in improving ADHD symptoms, in part by raising levels of dopamine and brain-derived neurotrophic factor (BDNF), two neurotransmitters responsible for growth and learning. In one 2011 study, a 28-day program of daily treadmill running, 30 minutes a day, raised levels of dopamine and BDNF in hyperactive rats and improved their ability to find their way around a complex maze.

In humans, exercise can temporarily raise levels of dopamine (and the adrenal hormone norepinephrine)—thus mimicking the effects of ADHD drugs like Ritalin and Adderall. In the brain, exercise can stimulate the prefrontal cortex, responsible for executive functioning, impulse control, and decision making, thus giving affected children more control and more time to evaluate moment-to-moment choices.

By heightening the senses, improving mood and focus, and relieving tension, exercise creates an ideal environment for a child to learn. At the same time, exercise improves neurogenesis—the building of new cells—which directly accelerates learning in itself.

Adults with ADHD should embrace any and all forms of exercise—pick one and run with it (literally). For kids, aerobic activity and structured activity involving teamwork and direct engagement with other kids is key. *Fun* should also be a leading determiner in your choice of activity: The more chances kids with ADHD have to feel good about themselves while exercising, the better and more effective it is in helping to alleviate their symptoms.

On a personal note, I don't have ADHD, but I can tell you from personal experience that exercising helps me focus my brain and makes me a better doctor. I discovered this in medical school. I had a much easier time studying and concentrating on the days I exercised. I carried this through to my residency as well, jumping rope at 3 a.m. in the on-call room. And it's still true for me today.

THE PROBLEM:
Depression

THE SYMPTOMS: You're down, unmotivated, uninterested. You may sleep or eat too much or too little; you may feel restless, anxious, and keyed up or, equally, tired, hopeless, and worn-out. Various physical problems, including digestive problems and aches and pains, may accompany these feelings.

WHAT'S GOING ON: Many cases of depression do in fact have a clear external cause. It may occur following a major life event such as divorce, the death of someone close to you, loss of a job, moving, or periods of intense stress. It may be symptomatic of menopause in women, low testosterone in men, a thyroid condition, or sleeping problems like apnea. People who work a swing shift, with no consistent pattern to their waking or sleeping hours, are especially prone to depression. And certain prescription drugs, including those for hepatitis C and beta-blockers for high blood pressure, can also cause depressive symptoms.

Depression can also come up for no apparent reason. Life can be pretty good and you can feel lousy anyway, losing interest in even enjoyable activities for weeks at a time. More than 2 weeks in a depressed state that has no clear external cause is known as major depressive disorder (MDD), or clinical depression.

Exercise is known as "nature's antidepressant," and lots of data shows why. One Norwegian study, for example, followed nearly 39,000 people from 2006–2008, so it's no small group. Individuals who reported moderate and high physical activity had significantly lower scores on depression and anxiety compared to the folks who did little or nothing.

Another study followed 2,000 people treated for congestive heart failure. In a year, the patients who exercised for 90 to 120 minutes a week saw greater reductions in depression symptoms than those who didn't.

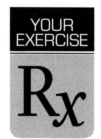

YOUR EXERCISE

GO FOR THE GOLD. Since exercise is "nature's antidepressant," use the gold standard of exercise in Part 3. Thirty minutes a day, at least 5 days a week, of moderate exercise like walking, or 30 minutes a day three times a week of heart-pumping aerobic activity has been shown to be very effective in fighting depression. As mentioned in Part 1, exercise may work *better* than antidepressant medications in some cases—without the negative side effects.

The longer-term effects of an exercise program on the symptoms of depression are less clear. But since 30 minutes of exercise brings on an immediate lift in mood, it may work as a motivator for a person who, by definition, doesn't feel motivated to do much of anything: I don't feel like exercising now, you can tell yourself, but after a half hour on this treadmill, I'll feel much better.

LIFT SOMETHING HEAVY.

Strength training has also been shown to be effective in easing depression, possibly because it enhances self-efficacy—or the feeling of having control over yourself and your environment. Many longtime lifters I've known have reflected on the one-to-one elegance of effort-to-results in their physical activity of choice: They enjoy the fact that they get out of the activity exactly what they put in.

When to Call a Doctor

Depression can become chronic and debilitating if untreated, so if you have symptoms without a clear external origin that persist for 2 weeks, you should consult your health care provider, who will help you come up with the course of treatment that will best suit you. That may include a combination of talk therapy, medication, and self-care measures like meditation.

Unless there's a compelling reason not to work out, however, any good treatment regimen for depression should include exercise: At the very least, it will help you maintain your fitness while you work your way through your symptoms. And it could provide a major key to your recovery.

THE PROBLEM:
Memory Loss and Cognition Problems

THE SYMPTOMS: Common symptoms of cognitive decline include an inability to focus, forgetting of names and dates, getting lost easily, repetition of the same thoughts, and difficulty with driving or other familiar tasks. Memory loss can come on as the result of an injury or other trauma, but more typically comes on gradually and often begins with a general decline in alertness.

WHAT'S GOING ON: Everyone experiences some decline in cognitive capacity as time progresses. These changes may begin as early as the midtwenties and include numerous changes to the physical structure of the brain itself as well as some of its functioning.

Aging is the primary cause of memory loss and a slowing or loss of cognitive powers; head trauma, depression, high blood pressure, and diabetes may also hasten the onset of these issues. Other risk factors include:

- **CHRONIC INFLAMMATION:** Often caused by smoking, obesity, poor sleep, and a poor diet, chronic inflammation may compromise the "blood-brain barrier," allowing inflammatory cytokines to enter the brain. *Cytokines* can damage and destroy existing neurons in the brain and impair the growth of new ones.

- **HORMONAL IMBALANCES:** Many hormones, including testosterone, estrogen, dehydroepiandrosterone (DHEA), pregnenolone, and thyroid hormones are involved in healthy cognition; imbalances can disrupt their healthy functioning.

- **CEREBROVASCULAR HEALTH:** Though it weighs only 3 pounds, your brain uses about 20 percent of the oxygen you breathe in. The carotid artery and its downstream tributaries are susceptible to *endothelial dysfunction,* the first step in atherosclerosis, or hardening of the arteries. Naturally, if the brain's blood supply is compromised so is cognition.

- **HDL (HIGH-DENSITY LIPOPROTEIN) LEVELS:** HDL is the "good" cholesterol because it shuttles cholesterol from your artery walls back to the liver for excretion. If HDL is low, this process slows down and greater buildup occurs. Low HDL has been linked with a decline in brain health, as well.

- **SOCIAL NETWORK AND CONNECTEDNESS:** The smaller your social network, the more likely you are to develop dementia; the more friends and connections you have, the less likely it is. Group activities, especially outdoors, have been shown to preserve brain health. And in case you're wondering, Facebook doesn't count.

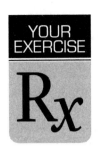

Can exercise really help with these problems? Yes, it can. Exercise, first and foremost, promotes better blood-flow to all areas of the body, including the brain. A brain with a good blood supply works better. And there's more: *Neuroplasticity*—the brain's ability to heal, grow, and change throughout life—is one of the more exciting concepts in exercise and medical science in the last 10 years or so. Essentially, science is telling us that you can teach old dogs new tricks—especially if those old dogs keep moving.

That's because exercise stimulates growth and adaptation in the brain, particularly around memory: A comprehensive review from 2007 indicated that both aerobic exercise and strength training improved cognitive functions in adults virtually across the board: memory, attention, decision making, multitasking, and planning all improved with exercise.

Other recent studies have centered on a protein called brain-derived neurotropic factor, or BDNF, which promotes health in nerve cells and contributes to memory. In one study, college men showed an uptick in BDNF levels—and higher scores on memory tests—following a half hour on an exercise bike (a control group who didn't exercise showed no such improvements).

Exercise appears to give brain functioning a short-term boost as well: In another test, a 4-week, four-times-a-week program of walking or jogging was shown to improve memory in sedentary adults, and people who exercised before the memory test got an even further memory boost. So if you've got a tough cognitive task coming up—a test, a job interview, a presentation—you might well kick your performance up a notch if you get yourself moving beforehand.

The bottom line? Exercise can absolutely improve both the structure and function of your brain, allowing you to stave off and even recover from age-related decline well into old age.

One final recommendation: Your brain will probably benefit even more from exercise and movement if you include some degree of novelty and variety in your program. Repetition of a familiar task doesn't seem to stimulate nearly the same brain growth as learning a new skill.

For the biggest improvements in memory and cognition, then, move in a *new* way: Learn to square dance, do tai chi, play tennis, do a martial art. Or, alternatively, simply hike a new trail, plant a new garden, change your cycling route. Such changes in routine can be small, but your brain will thank you for making them.

When to Call a Doctor

Dementia isn't always caused by Alzheimer's disease (they're actually distinct conditions), but you should check with a doctor if you or a loved one seems to be having frequent episodes of confusion, disorientation, and memory loss that interferes with daily living.

THE PROBLEM:
Chronic Stress

THE SYMPTOMS: Feelings of anxiety, overwhelming pressure, and lack of control. A person experiencing chronic stress may have digestive problems, sweaty palms, an increased resting heart and respiratory rate, shortness of breath, and cold hands and feet. Over time, stress may lead to depression, fatigue, frequent headaches, backaches, and other signs of physical tension. Weight loss or gain may also result.

WHAT'S GOING ON: In today's world, information and demands related to that information come at us from every direction, every screen, all the time. You feel like there's no escape. And you're not alone—millions of people share these feelings. And chronic stress takes a toll.

Stress, on its own, is like fire: When it's contained, it can be a big help, motivating you to stay focused and on task. When it's out of control, however, it's a big problem.

Psychologists call the state of optimal stress *eustress*—an in-the-groove feeling in which external demands match your ability to handle them. When an emergency or demanding situation comes up unexpectedly, you may also experience acute stress—a sudden "switching on" of the stress response that helps you rise to the occasion and handle a possible threat.

Often, though, the daily stresses of life pile up and spiral out of control, leading to a chronic state of emotional and physical arousal: Work projects are due, the mortgage is late, the kids need braces, and *whammo*—you feel like the walls are closing in. Major life events such as divorce, death, moving, loss of a job, or financial hardship can be triggers.

This unpleasant sensation is technically called *hyperstress:* the feeling that you are unable to meet the demands being placed on you. If the situation remains unchanged, hyperstress may evolve into *chronic stress.*

The symptoms of excessive stress are caused by activation of the sympathetic nervous system, which prepares us for physical action—flight or fight—when we encounter a threat, and by cortisol, the major stress hormone, which helps regulate energy and can cue the body to store fat. Chronically elevated cortisol can thus lead to sleep disruptions, food cravings, increased appetite, and obesity.

Hypostress, in which circumstances are insufficiently challenging to engage you, is another type of stress. People trapped in repetitive jobs often experience this type of stress, which can lead a person to feel uninspired, restless, irritable, and, ultimately, depressed.

It's hard to go through life without at least some periods of unpleasant stress; the trick is to find ways to manage and control it as much as possible.

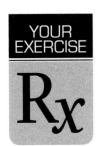

YOUR EXERCISE

Rx

Exercise can be very effective in helping you prevent and overcome the symptoms of stress. Vigorous exercise busies the brain and gives it a break from mulling over the stressful situation. Exercise also causes cortisol levels to drop acutely, reducing symptoms of anxiety and restlessness and helping you to focus. If stress is affecting sleep, regular exercise can also help restore the normal circadian cycle, leading to better sleep at night and more focus during the day.

Some hard-charging, stressed-out types engage in physical activities they feel they *should* do for their health or appearance. Exercise can thus become another obligation on a never-ending to-do list. So select a form of exercise based on preference and enjoyment.

The workouts in Part 3 are a great place to start. Also consider the following recommendations:

• **TAKE A BREATH.** According to the American College of Sports Medicine, exercise modalities that include attention to breathing—yoga, tai chi, Feldenkrais, and Pilates, among others—may be particularly helpful in relieving the symptoms of stress, as focus on breath helps slow respiration and heart rate. (See "Blow Away Stress," on page 42, for an easy-to-learn, 1-minute stress-buster based on the yoga sun salutation.)

• **GO AEROBIC.** A 2008 study indicated that a lunchtime aerobics class lasting from 45 to 60 minutes was an effective stress reducer, improving the mood and focus of white-collar workers, as well as the ability to get along with their coworkers. The mood-boosting effects of exercise only accrued on days when the workers exercised—so when you're facing a challenging day, it may be all the *more* important to get that workout in.

• **GO OUTSIDE.** If the weather cooperates, exercising outdoors may be more effective in reducing stress than working out in a gym. A 2011 review of studies published in *Environmental Science and Technology* found that people who exercised outdoors experienced "greater feelings of revitalization, increased energy, and positive engagement, together with decreases in tension, confusion, anger, and depression," compared with people who exercised indoors.

When to Call a Doctor

If there's no end in sight to stress, you may have to make a major life change. Call a health care provider if

• You have experienced a marked decline in work or school performance

• You have irrational fears

• You feel unable to cope with the demands of your daily life

• You misuse alcohol or drugs

• You experience major, unexplained changes in your sleeping or eating habits

• You have suicidal thoughts or urges to hurt others

• You engage in self-mutilation or other self-destructive or dangerous behavior

• You have a sustained withdrawn mood

THE PROBLEM:
Fatigue

THE SYMPTOMS: Your mojo's all but gone: You're weary, unmotivated, drained of energy. Fatigue may or may not result in drowsiness—the urge to sleep.

WHAT'S GOING ON: We've all been tired. Fatigue is normal following physical exertion, periods of high stress, boredom, sleep deprivation, or jet lag. It's not serious, and it's usually relieved by a good night's sleep, a healthy meal or two, and a return to normal daily rhythms.

However, unexplained fatigue can sometimes be a symptom of a more serious underlying condition, such as anemia, cancer, diabetes, congestive heart failure, fibromyalgia, kidney and liver disease, and high or low thyroid. It can also be a side effect of anorexia, depression, malnutrition, and certain medications, including antidepressants, sleep aids, antihistamines, steroids, and diuretics.

If you feel continuously fatigued for 6 months or more, and all other possible causes are ruled out, you may receive a diagnosis of chronic fatigue syndrome (CFS), which often begins with flu-like symptoms and morphs into a state of severe and continuous lethargy that is only minimally relieved by rest and sleep. CFS is by no means fully understood but may be related to a number of other factors, including anemia, environmental allergies, sleep disorders, psychiatric or neurological problems, hormonal dysfunction, and low blood pressure. As many as 1 million adults have CFS, mostly women between the ages of 20 and 40.

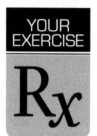

YOUR EXERCISE Rx

Throwing yourself into a full-out, sweat-pouring workout to relieve your symptoms of fatigue may seem counterintuitive; it's probably the last thing you want to do when you're tired. But research shows that you probably don't have to: A 2008 study published in the Swiss medical journal *Psychotherapy and Psychosomatics* found that low- *or* moderate-intensity exercise (20 minutes at a stretch) resulted in a 20 percent increase in energy levels after 6 weeks. Also, low-intensity exercisers reported a 65 percent drop in fatigue symptoms, as opposed to moderate exercisers who reported only a 49 percent drop. So if you're experiencing fatigue, go for a walk, but don't go for a sprint. Make it a day when you stay well within your capabilities.

Exercise can also help relieve fatigue symptoms associated with chronic conditions like cancer and fibromyalgia, though again, you should take care to keep intensity levels in check: A review of studies stated that prescribing exercise for people with fibromyalgia required "finesse," as too little could have no effect and too much could exacerbate symptoms. Mild aerobic training, strength training, tai chi, and yoga were all found to be beneficial for relieving symptoms of fatigue.

The upshot? When you're fatigued, a little exercise goes a long way. The toughest part here is taking those first few steps out the door. But once you get going, you'll feel *so* much better. Just commit to the first 5 minutes and watch what happens.

When to Call a Doctor

If you have chronic fatigue that isn't relieved by exercise or other positive lifestyle changes, see a doctor for the reasons stated in the "What's Going On" section: Fatigue can be a side effect of a host of health problems. Exercise may help, but you need a doctor's help to pinpoint a more severe problem.

THE PROBLEM:
Low Self-Esteem

THE SYMPTOMS: This is a tough one to define, but low self-esteem affects almost everyone at some point in their lives. You may feel general dissatisfaction; feelings of worthlessness; hypersensitivity to criticism; chronic indecision and fear of mistakes; excessive desire to please others; perfectionism; guilt over past mistakes, regardless of how small; defensiveness; negativity; envy.

WHAT'S GOING ON: Low self-esteem can be "state" or "trait" in nature: Your self-esteem can be chronically low, or it can plummet as the result of a specific event. To some extent, a waxing or waning of self-esteem is just part of life's fascinating and exasperating ride: Sometimes you're up, sometimes you're down. But chronically low self-esteem can be crippling for some people, keeping you from enjoying your life or trying anything challenging, new, or exciting.

It's possible that chronic feelings of low self-esteem can be an extension of another psychological disorder such as depression, anxiety disorder, or others. On the other hand, low self-esteem could simply be a product of self-doubt, shyness, or a general lack of confidence.

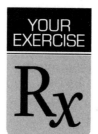

YOUR EXERCISE Rx

Your fifth-grade gym teacher was at least half right: Exercise *can* boost self-esteem. A 2012 study in Perspectives in Public Health showed that exercise had positive effects on self-esteem and mood in both the short- and long-term. Participants reported positive boosts after individual workouts, as well as broader improvements over a 6-week period. Exercising outdoors may help even more: Folks who did countryside and urban park walks had the best results.

As always, the safe choice is something aerobic and of moderate intensity that you perform for around a half hour. Repetitive, easy movements can help relieve anxiety, tension, anger, and fatigue and get you back on track emotionally. Swimming and cycling score high marks in studies. Also making a strong showing are easier and more therapeutic forms of movement like yoga, tai chi, and qigong.

One 2009 study suggested that people who engaged in high-intensity anaerobic activity actually felt *more* anxious following exercise. However, the subjects were first-timers and only completed the workouts once. If you're an avid strength-trainer, chances are the weights make you feel effective and strong—so by all means, go ahead and hit the dumbbells, and hit 'em hard, if you need a boost.

The upshot is to let enjoyment be your guide.

When to Call a Doctor

If intense feelings of worthlessness and apathy persist for at least 2 weeks, you could be dealing with depression or other mental health issues. These types of problems can be chronic and debilitating if left untreated. A doctor may refer you to a therapist or other mental health care provider.

BLOW AWAY STRESS

You're stressed out, overworked, wrung out. There's no energy—much less time—for a real workout, but you need to get yourself calm and focused fast. What do you do? The easy answer is *breathe*.

For centuries, pro athletes, politicians, and other high-stakes performers have relied on movement-based breathing exercises, along with stretching movements, to steady their nerves when the pressure's on. Now you can, too.

Studies have shown that mind-body practices like yoga, tai chi, the Feldenkrais Method, Pilates, and other systems can be very effective in relieving stress and anxiety. So if you're starting to feel an avalanche of obligations piling up, take 1 minute to perform the following stretch-and-relax drill, based on the yoga sun salutation. Repeat the cycle up to five times, depending on available time. Afterward you should feel calmer and more centered.

1. Find a quiet place where you won't be disturbed for 5 minutes. Turn off the phone, computer, alarms of any kind, and anything distracting. It may also be helpful to dim the lights.

2. Stand erect with your feet together, looking straight ahead.

3. Inhale deeply and simultaneously reach both hands directly overhead. If possible, press your palms together.

4. Exhale fully, and simultaneously bend forward at your hip joint, reaching your hands toward the floor, assuming a "forward bend" posture.

5. Inhale deeply, and simultaneously step backward with your right foot, keeping the knee straight. Look forward, place your hands on the floor on either side of your left leg, and sink into a deep lunge.

6. Exhale fully and simultaneously step your left leg back so your feet are side by side. Lift your hips high in the air, straighten your arms and legs, and pressing your chest down toward the floor, assume a down-dog pose.

7. Inhale deeply and simultaneously bend your arms, dive-bombing your upper body forward, swooping down toward the floor and then upward again, straightening your arms, arching your back and coming into the cobra pose.

8. Exhale and return to the down-dog posture.

9. Inhale deeply and step forward with your right foot, coming into a deep lunge on your right side.

10. Exhale fully and step forward with your left foot, coming back to the forward bend pose.

11. Inhale deeply and stand again, reaching your hands overhead again, palms together.

12. Exhale fully as you bring your hands downward into a prayer position, in front of your chest.

THE PROBLEM:
Sleep Apnea

THE SYMPTOMS: Repeated, chronic interruptions in normal breathing patterns during sleep, lasting from a few seconds to a minute or more, caused either by an obstruction in the airway (obstructed sleep apnea, OSA), a lack of breathing effort (central sleep apnea, CSA), or both. Side effects of sleep apnea include fatigue, vision problems, irritability, possible weight gain, high blood pressure, and difficulty concentrating.

WHAT'S GOING ON: Deep sleep causes the muscles around your airways to relax and, depending on the position of the sleeper and the structure of the soft tissues in the throat, causes obstruction in the airways, cutting off the breath. The same structures that cause apnea can also cause snoring—another common side effect of the condition.

Sleep apnea is fairly common, particularly among overweight people, but often goes unnoticed, as interruptions in nighttime breathing usually cause sleep disruption but do not cause the person to wake up fully. Sleep apnea can therefore remain undiagnosed for years, until the more obvious side effects of chronic sleep deprivation start to become obvious or until someone else notices the breathing pauses—which often show up as pauses in the person's snoring.

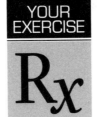
YOUR EXERCISE Rx

Exercise and sleep can work wonders together. A good night's sleep can help you have a stronger workout. A stronger workout can improve your sleep quality. And a majority of the positive physical recovery from exercise happens while you sleep. As important as exercise is, sleep is the most important activity of your day. That's why it's imperative to use exercise to get the best night's sleep you can.

Obesity is the primary risk factor for sleep apnea—and the most changeable—so the number-one general-health priority for people with sleep apnea should be weight loss. Exercise combined with smart eating is the fastest road to weight loss. Numerous studies have shown improvements—and some, complete alleviation of apnea symptoms—with a combination of exercise and a low-calorie diet. One study, published in the journal *Sleep* in 2011, indicated that exercise may help to lessen mild symptoms even without any weight loss.

See Parts 3 and 4 for some effective, fast weight-loss workout and diet tips.

When to Call a Doctor

If a loved one notices that your breathing stops repeatedly at night, and you are experiencing unexplained fatigue during the day, see a doctor. They may set up a sleep study to monitor you in a lab overnight and to make an accurate diagnosis. If you have sleep apnea, your health care provider can supply you with a device that can help keep your airway clear at night. Though these devices can be uncomfortable, and weight loss is probably a more practical course of treatment.

THE PROBLEM:
Poor Sleep Quality

THE SYMPTOMS: Fatigue, lethargy, and lack of motivation; weight gain; increased risk of diabetes, heart disease, and other health problems; moodiness and irritability; reduced creativity and problem-solving skills; inability to cope with stress; frequent colds and infections; impaired motor skills and increased risk of accidents; difficulty making decisions.

WHAT'S GOING ON: Among the three major habits that can ensure good health, sleep probably gets ignored most frequently. We understand we're supposed to eat well and exercise, and at the very least we probably feel a little guilty when we don't. Skimping on sleep is another matter: Most people who do it regularly—and research suggests that 25 percent of Americans fall into that category (I think the number's much higher)—just consider it an inevitable side effect of a busy life.

But chronic sleep deprivation is sneaky: It may feel so normal to you that you don't realize the damage you're causing, inside or outside, or how much your day-to-day effectiveness could improve if you got more sleep.

There are four stages of sleep.

The first two are transition phases from wakefulness and typically take just a few minutes each. During deep sleep, the third, "can't wake you with a foghorn" phase, your body releases growth hormone, builds new muscle, and repairs damages caused by stress. REM sleep, a lighter phase during which you dream, seems to improve learning and cognition: People learning new mental skills have trouble recalling them if deprived of this phase of sleep.

During the night, one pass through these four stages takes roughly 90 minutes, and the cycle repeats four to six times per night. The amount of time you spend in each phase shifts as the night goes on: Most people rack up more deep sleep at the beginning of the night and more REM sleep closer to morning. Staying up late, then, tends to deprive you of deep sleep, whereas rising early can cut down on REM time.

Sleep deprivation can also affect appetite and metabolism, leading to overeating and, over time, weight gain and obesity.

Anything less than 7.5 to 9 hours of sleep can throw your game off both physically and mentally. But the quality of sleep is often just as important as the quantity: Some people seem to spend enough time in the sack but don't feel rested during the day. That may be due to a chronic condition like sleep apnea (see page 43), or it may be a combination of other factors including:

- Stress and anxiety

- Loud noises, including crying children and loud neighbors

- Pain

- Late-night consumption of alcohol or caffeine

- GERD (gastroesophageal reflux disorder)

- Certain medicines, including steroids, beta-blockers, and pain medications

- The herbal supplements ginseng and guarana

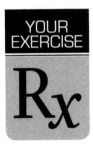

YOUR EXERCISE Rx

Exercise is a terrific sleep aid. One 2011 study found that regular aerobic workouts significantly improved sleep quality among people with insomnia, while also alleviating feelings of depression and anxiety, improving mood and increasing daytime alertness. Meditative, calming practices like yoga and tai chi have also been shown to improve sleep quality.

For best results, it may be useful to train shortly after waking: One study compared the sleep habits of morning, afternoon, and evening exercisers and found that those who worked out in the morning saw the biggest improvements in sleep quality.

I personally prefer a morning workout. Some research suggests that morning exercise raises your metabolism for the rest of the day. But be realistic. If lunchtime is the most convenient time for you to work out, do it. An evening exerciser? Go forth and sweat. One thing to keep in mind, however: Try to wrap up your exercise 2 to 3 hours before you go to bed to give your body time to wind down.

As far as what kind of exercise to do, take your pick. A good, healthy sweat for 30 minutes a day—from any activity—is enough to do the trick. See Part 3 of the book for dozens of ideas.

When to Call a Doctor

Chronic insomnia—difficulty falling and staying asleep even when you do get to bed at a reasonable hour—is a serious matter. If you're consistently fatigued and feel that lack of good sleep is cutting into your daily activities, a doctor will help you determine if your difficulties sleeping are caused by sleep apnea, a digestive issue like GERD, anxiety, or some other treatable condition, and take appropriate action. You may need to stay overnight in a sleep lab for observation.

CHAPTER 2

Cardiopulmonary Problems

We're aerobic creatures.

That doesn't mean that all of us like to don off-the-shoulder sweatshirts and leg warmers and hit step classes (though maybe we'd all be healthier if we did!). It just means that we use a lot of oxygen, whether we're pushing ourselves to the max on the elliptical machine or lying in a hammock with an iPad. The vast majority of processes in our bodies—from running to digesting to breathing and even thinking—require oxygen, and plenty of it. So the cardiopulmonary system is pretty important. If it stops working, so do you.

On the other hand, the better it functions, the better *you* function. Having a condition like asthma, high blood pressure, or heart disease can make exercise challenging—but hardly impossible. The good news? Exercise is precisely the thing that will improve all these problems. The data on cardiopulmonary disease is among the strongest we have.

THE PROBLEM:
Asthma

THE SYMPTOMS: Recurrent coughing, wheezing, shortness of breath, a feeling of tightness in the chest, and difficulty breathing.

WHAT'S GOING ON: Asthma is an inflammatory condition for which there is no cure and whose causes are not entirely known—though both genetic and environmental factors seem to be at work. You're more likely to have asthma if one or both parents do, and most people's symptoms get worse in the presence of specific external triggers, which vary from person to person. Common triggers include allergens like dust and mold, tobacco, perfumes, or emotional and psychological stress.

Interestingly, a surprising number of athletes, particularly in endurance sports, suffer from *exercise-induced bronchospasm*—a condition usually controlled with the use of a fast-acting inhaler.

Asthma varies significantly in severity from one person to another. For some, symptoms are chronic and only minimally responsive to drugs; for others, they're intermittent, have a clear cause, and are controlled very effectively by drugs.

Gaining weight tends to worsen, and in some cases bring on, symptoms of asthma, perhaps because fat cells can lead to a "proinflammatory" state throughout the body.

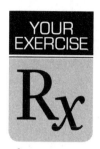 **YOUR EXERCISE**

It wasn't too long ago that overprotective parents would lock their asthmatic kids indoors and prevent them from exercising at all. Unfortunately, lack of activity can lead to a vicious cycle in which the child (or adult) moves less, gains weight, and sees a worsening of symptoms.

These days, health care providers recommend that people with asthma *do* exercise, not only for all the usual health benefits it provides, but as a way of helping to manage asthma symptoms: Results from a 2012 review of studies suggested that the fitter your cardiovascular system, the less debilitating the effects of the disease. Research also shows that athletes with exercise-induced asthma often find that their symptoms diminish as they become more fit.

Any type of exercise that interests you—cardio or strength training, outdoor and indoor sports—is fine. See the workouts in Part 3 for any number of exercise combinations that are both challenging and diverse. You won't be bored.

However, people with asthma may need to take the following extra precautions:

• Keep up with dosages of all prescription medications and other protocols recommended by your doctor.

- Take a fast-acting rescue inhaler 15 minutes before exercising, and keep it handy during exercise.

- For those with exercise-induced asthma, avoid working out in cold weather. Introducing cold, dry air to your lungs quickly can trigger an attack.

- A proper warmup for 10 minutes can also help prepare your lungs for a workout. Build up to full effort slowly to prevent a sudden shock to your lungs.

- Also avoid environmental triggers during workouts: High humidity, car exhaust, smog, grass, and other outdoor irritants may worsen symptoms. Some triggers are seasonal, so you may need to avoid certain areas at certain times of year.

- If necessary, exercise indoors.

- Pay particular attention to warming up and cooling down, as a sudden change in intensity of movement may trigger an episode.

Children with asthma often see a reduction in symptoms in adolescence due to growth in the bronchial pathways. Sometimes symptoms disappear completely. Parents can take advantage of this window by encouraging vigorous aerobic and anaerobic exercise— taking the precautions listed above—starting when their child is about 12 or 13. Lifetime lung capacity and pulmonary function are largely determined during this period of growth, so the more you develop as an adolescent, the more you'll have in the years that follow.

When to Call a Doctor

If you have an asthma episode, see your doctor. He or she will most likely prescribe a fast-acting inhaler for acute symptoms, and possibly a longer-acting inhaled corticosteroid as well. The drugs are easy to take, have few side effects, and are, in general, very effective. If you ignore it, asthma can be serious, but with the right treatment, it doesn't have to slow you down.

THE SYMPTOMS: Some people with cardiovascular disease experience obvious side effects, including shortness of breath, chest pains, tightness in the jaw, pain across the shoulders or back, or discomfort in either arm. Often, however, these conditions—which don't just affect the heart—have silent symptoms and are only detectable through testing.

WHAT'S GOING ON: Cardiovascular diseases, including diseases of the heart or blood vessels, vascular diseases of the brain and kidney, and peripheral arterial disease, are the leading cause of death worldwide.

In the case of coronary heart disease (CHD), one of the most common forms of cardiovascular disease, calcium and cholesterol form plaque deposits inside the coronary arteries of the heart, limiting the blood and oxygen that the heart receives.

During a cerebrovascular accident (CVA, or stroke), blood supply to the brain is cut off due to ischemia (lack of bloodflow), blockage (arterial embolism, thrombosis), or leakage (hemorrhage), sometimes causing permanent damage to physical functioning.

Some other common types of cardiovascular disease include angina pectoris (chest pain), congestive heart failure, cardiomyopathy (which covers diseases of the heart muscle), and hypertensive heart disease, or diseases associated with high blood pressure.

That's one frightening list. Deadly as they are, it's possible to manage— or at least mitigate—nearly all the risk factors associated with cardiovascular diseases. Some combination of high blood pressure, obesity, lack of physical activity, elevated cholesterol, smoking, and excessive drinking accounts for the majority of cases of cardiovascular disease. Other factors like age, family history, diabetes, and gender (men are more susceptible) also increase your risk.

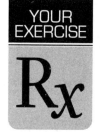

YOUR EXERCISE Smart exercise substantially reduces your risk of cardiovascular disease, and thereby increases your chances of living a long and healthy life. Many studies have shown this, but one of the biggest of its kind, the Framingham Heart Study, has shown definitively that regular, long-term physical exertion protects against death from cardiovascular disease. In 1948, researchers signed up more than 5,200 people and followed them for decades. In 1971, 5,100 of those folk's children were signed up and followed. In 2002, a third generation was added and the study continues to this day. Safe to say, it's authoritative, and similar results have been found in studies worldwide. A recent one published in the *Asian Journal of Sports Medicine* found that Iranian women who walked on a treadmill three times a week for 30 minutes at 70 to 80 percent of their maximum heart rate significantly lowered their 10-year risk for coronary heart disease after just 12 weeks on the program. In people who have already had heart attacks, exercise can lower the risk of dying from a future event by up to 25 percent.

In order to be helpful, however, an exercise routine needs to be *routine*—a predicable regimen performed frequently, preferably every day. In people with increased cardiovascular risk who are normally sedentary, sudden, vigorous exertion can be dangerous. During winter months, for example, emergency rooms are often inundated with middle-aged and older men who have had heart attacks while shoveling snow. So avoid vigorous stop-and-go activities, particularly when just starting an exercise program, and be aware of the warning signs (see "The Symptoms" on the opposite page).

Without specific recommendations from a doctor, however, guidelines for exercise for a person with cardiovascular disease, or at risk for developing it, should be the same as for the general population: Thirty minutes of moderate aerobic activity on 3 or more days per week and 30 minutes of strength training on 2 or more days per week. The American Heart Association also suggests that increasing daily physical activity outside of formal exercise—taking walking breaks, gardening, and doing housework, for example—can be helpful in preventing cardiovascular disease as well.

I also suggest setting a fitness goal—something that will keep you not just exercising, but striving to improve your fitness as you train. That's one of the most gratifying ways to approach exercise.

IMPORTANT NOTE: See page 54 for a special section on exercising after a heart attack or heart disease diagnosis. It's some of the most important information in this book.

When to Call a Doctor

Head to the ER at any sign of symptoms (listed on the opposite page). Cardiovascular disease is serious business, and you should work with a doctor to help manage your symptoms through lifestyle changes like diet and exercise, the use of medication, or both. See page 54 for important information on exercise and a heart disease diagnosis.

THE PROBLEM:
High Blood Pressure (Hypertension)

THE SYMPTOMS: Sometimes called "the silent killer," high blood pressure often has no noticeable symptoms. Anything above a reading of 120/80 (systolic over diastolic pressure, measured from a seated position in milligrams of mercury) is considered prehypertensive. If your systolic pressure is 140 or more or your diastolic pressure is 90 or more, as measured on two separate occasions, your blood pressure is considered high.

Occasionally, very high blood pressure (diastolic pressure of 110 or more), also called *malignant hypertension*, may result in more obvious symptoms, including headaches, dizziness, blurred vision, nausea and vomiting, chest pain, and shortness of breath. A person with malignant hypertension should seek immediate medical care.

WHAT'S GOING ON: Blood pressure is a measure of the force of your blood pushing against the walls of your arteries as your blood pumps. Systolic pressure—the number on top—measures that force as your heart beats; diastolic pressure, the number on the bottom, measures that force between beats. Of the 75 million Americans with high blood pressure 30 percent are unaware that they have it—which is why it's important to have yours screened regularly.

Although you usually can't feel it, hypertension is associated with a host of nasty health outcomes that you definitely want to avoid, including damage to blood vessels in the eyes, thickening of the heart muscle, heart attacks, hardening of the arteries, kidney failure, and strokes.

The causes for high blood pressure aren't entirely understood, but research shows that your risk is affected by some factors largely out of your control, including:

- **GENDER** (men have higher blood pressure than women)

- **AGE** (due to a hardening of the arteries, or *arteriosclerosis*)

- **FAMILY HISTORY** of cardiovascular disease

- **EMOTIONAL STATE**

- **TIME OF DAY**

- **ETHNICITY** (blood pressure tends to be higher among African Americans and other minorities)

- **SOCIOECONOMIC STATUS** (lower-income and less-educated people are more susceptible to high blood pressure)

However, blood pressure is equally affected by your daily lifestyle choices: Being overweight, obese, and sedentary drives up blood pressure considerably, as does consuming excessive alcohol, saturated fats, trans fats, and, in some cases, salt. Another factor in elevated BP: *lack of exercise.*

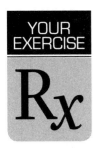

YOUR EXERCISE

R𝑥

In most people, though not all, blood pressure is very responsive to exercise. According to one study, a single session of aerobic exercise (40 minutes on a stationary bike) lowered blood pressure for a full 24 hours in people with hypertension. Exercising daily, then, can have a significant impact on average blood pressure and may eliminate symptoms altogether. On average, regular exercise causes both systolic and diastolic blood pressure to drop by 5 to 10 points. Any weight you lose from exercise will also improve your blood pressure readings.

As long as you have been cleared for physical activity, the American College of Sports Medicine recommends combining moderate aerobic exercise, 30 minutes at least three times a week, with resistance training at least twice a week, for reductions in blood pressure. Swimming workouts, as well as faster, more intense cardiovascular workouts, in the form of sprint-style interval training, have also shown to be effective, but check with your doctor to see which type of training, and at what intensity level, is best for you. See the workouts in Part 3 for a host of ideas.

BONUS IDEAS: Consuming certain foods—low-fat dairy products for calcium, fruits and vegetables, plenty of potassium (abundant in white potatoes, soybeans, and bananas), and even small amounts of dark chocolate—can also help improve blood pressure.

When to Call a Doctor

If you experience any of the symptoms of malignant hypertension—chest pain, shortness of breath, nausea, dizziness, or blurred vision—go to the ER immediately.

Your doctor should help you monitor and manage milder hypertension symptoms. He or she may give you advice on diet and exercise and, if that does not clear up your problem, may prescribe medication (60 percent of people with high blood pressure take medication for the condition). Some of the treatments your doctor may prescribe include diuretics, beta-blockers, calcium channel blockers, and angiotensin-converting enzymes (ACE), some of which require that you stay on them for life.

SPECIAL SECTION
Exercising with Heart Disease

You already know that heart disease is the number one killer on the planet.

At some point, you or someone close to you will have a heart disease diagnosis. It could come from a routine physical. Or it could come from a sudden cardiac event, like a heart attack. It doesn't really matter how the diagnosis comes—when it does, it's the most frightening thing you'll ever hear.

But I want you to listen carefully: I don't care if you're scared. You must exercise. A workout might seem like the most impossible thing to try after you've been diagnosed with heart disease or had a heart attack. But it's vital.

Think about it this way: Even after a heart attack or heart disease diagnosis, your heart is *still* a muscle, it will *still* grow stronger from exercise, and you'll *still* have a lesser chance of a cardiac event than if you didn't exercise. Furthermore, the exercise will *still* help your blood pressure, cholesterol, and weight.

Research has backed this up, as heart attack survivors who exercise don't have to take as much medication, require fewer major surgeries like bypasses, and are less likely to die from a second heart attack than those who stay on the couch.

You'd be crazy not to exercise with heart disease.

Here are some ideas of how you can, and what to expect . . .

THE NAME OF THE GAME? SAFETY

If you've been diagnosed with cardiovascular disease, work with your doctor to set up a smart and, most importantly, safe exercise plan. Your doctor, knowing your individual condition, will be able to guide you on what exercises you can attempt and how hard you should push. If you've survived a heart attack, you'll most likely be working with a cardiac rehabilitation team at first to get moving again. They'll supervise your activity for several weeks or months, depending on what's needed.

EMBRACE:

• **Having Fun.** Exercise should be enjoyable—do something you love.

• **Stretching,** especially before a workout. See the Dynamic Warmup starting on page 180.

• **Traditional Cardio.** Walking, jogging, biking, swimming, etc. These activities help your body get better at using oxygen, and they work your heart.

- **Strength Training** (aka resistance training). Building muscle will make every activity easier.

IMPORTANT NOTE: People with heart failure should avoid certain resistance exercises, particularly isometric moves that force your muscle to work against an immovable object (pushups, for example).

- **Hydration.** Your body runs on water. Your urine should always look like light lemonade.

AVOID:

- **Heavy Lifting.** Consult your doctor about lifting or pushing heavy objects. This means weights, but also other things like snow shoveling, raking and hauling leaves, digging, etc.

- **Extreme Outdoor Temperatures.** Cold or hot, humid weather can affect your breathing, circulation, and sweat rate.

- **Saunas and Steam Baths,** for the same reasons.

- **Geographic Areas** that could make you overexert yourself, such as steep hills.

- **Exercising if You Feel Sick** or have a fever. Wait several days until after your symptoms disappear before resuming activity (it's worth consulting your doctor about this).

HOW HARD SHOULD YOU EXERCISE?

Again, this is something to consult your doctor about, but as every person has different fitness levels, in general it's smart to consult a Rated Perceived Exertion Scale (see chart). It's a simple self-evaluation scale numbered between 0 and 10. During any activity, ask yourself, "How hard am I working?" and assign a number.

A safe range would be between 3 and 4—high enough to get a good workout but not so high that you end up exhausting yourself. If you need rest during the workout, take it. But always try to finish—that's how you get stronger.

THE RATED PERCEIVED EXERTION SCALE

0	Nothing
0.5	Barely noticeable
1	Very light
2	Light
3	Moderate
4	Somewhat heavy
5–6	Heavy
7–9	Very heavy
10	100 percent full effort

For a more accurate reading of your effort during exercise, your doctor may recommend you use a heart rate monitor and keep your heart rate within a certain range of your maximum heart rate. To calculate your max heart rate, subtract your age from 220. If you shoot for the 3 to 4 range on the Rated Perceived Exertion Scale, you'll want to keep your heart rate at roughly 70 percent of your max rate.

For example, if you're 50, your max heart rate is 170. Seventy percent of 170 is 119 beats per minute.

To give you an idea why 70 percent is your target, that equates to a light-to-moderate intensity level during exercise. Sixty percent of your max would be considered "light." Approach 80 percent, or higher, and you're looking at "hard."

So that heart rate monitor can be a handy thing.

Stop exercising if you feel any of the following:

- Shortness of breath

- Rapid or irregular heartbeat (If you still have an elevated heart rate after 15 minutes of rest, 120–150 beats per minute, seek medical help and alert your doctor.)

- Chest pain

- Pressure in the neck, arm, jaw, or shoulder

- Weak

- Dizzy or lightheaded

IS ENDURANCE EXERCISE DANGEROUS FOR THE HEART?

Every once in a while you'll hear about someone, or know someone personally, who has a sudden heart attack during or after a long run. It's always shocking, but even more so because "[INSERT NAME HERE] was so healthy! How can someone who is in such great shape have a heart attack?"

Unfortunately, the answer is pretty simple: Heart disease can happen to anyone, even the most fit among us. Lifestyle is a huge factor in who gets heart disease, but it's also a scientific fact that genetics play a part, as well. Someone could be superfit but be genetically predetermined for heart disease because of family history. And who knows? Maybe that person's terrific fitness kept the disease at bay for a much longer period than if he or she was sedentary. You just never know.

Situations like this make some people ask (usually in frustration), "What's the point of exercising if I'm doomed anyway?"

My answer (trying to resist my own frustration): Healthier life! Longer life! Higher quality of life!

My overall message here is that studies on the benefits of exercise are far more compelling than studies that cite running and endurance sports as dangerous. And even if heart disease does strike, the higher your fitness is, the higher your chances are of surviving an event, and the faster your recovery will be.

If you think you're a candidate for a heart attack, here's my message:

- Exercise regularly
- See your doctor annually
- Listen to your body continuously

If you feel shortness of breath, dizziness, or faint during exercise, make sure you see your doctor before charging ahead. Exercise is medicine, but you need to be smart about how you administer it.

CHAPTER 3

Metabolic Problems

Your metabolism is ground zero for the war on fat.

If you're interested in losing weight, trimming fat, or just keeping the leanness you already have, then maintaining the speed, functioning, and efficiency of your metabolism should be your primary health focus.

Metabolism is the sum total of all the chemical reactions going on in your body at any point, and it includes both *anabolic* reactions, which result in the building of tissues such as bone and muscle mass, and *catabolic* reactions, in which tissues are broken down. Anabolic and catabolic reactions happen in your body every second: Old tissue dies off, new tissue is built. Day to day, these millions of building-and-destroying reactions more or less balance each other out, guided by the body's natural tendency toward equilibrium, or *homeostasis*.

Metabolic problems, like the accumulation of visceral fat and the now-common group of symptoms we call metabolic syndrome, are examples of how that balance can shift for the worse, causing metabolism to slow, fat to accumulate, and health in general to decline. Through consistent exercise and a smart diet, however, you can shift the balance the other way, too, setting your metabolic dial for catabolizing, rather than accumulating, fat, and for adding muscle mass at the same time. Keep it up and the new homeostasis can be a newly lean and muscular you.

THE PROBLEM:
Type 2 Diabetes (Diabetes Mellitus Type 2) and Hyperglycemia

THE SYMPTOMS: Excessive thirst, frequent urination, constant hunger, and fatigue. Blurred vision, weight gain, numbness in the hands or feet, itchiness, erectile dysfunction, and in women, recurrent vaginal infections may also occur.

WHAT'S GOING ON: People with diabetes can't process food energy properly. In healthy people, the hormone insulin, made in the pancreas, helps metabolize the carbohydrates you eat into usable energy. In people with type 2 diabetes, the body becomes unresponsive to insulin and therefore unable to process sugar. This creates a "bottleneck" of unused glucose in your bloodstream—and blood sugar rises precipitously, a state known as *hyperglycemia*. Glucose, for all its wonderful properties, is also corrosive to your body's tissue if it stays around too long. That's why you have a big insulin spike when you eat something sweet—your body is trying to clear the excess glucose from your blood as quickly as possible. That's also why a high-sugar, high-carb diet can lead to type 2 diabetes: Your body jacks up the insulin production to take care of the sugar and your insulin

receptors become less sensitive, which requires more insulin to get the job done. A nasty cycle ensues, with your pancreas eventually pooping out because it can't keep up with the constantly increasing insulin demands.

Since your body's cells are unable to use the energy available, you may start to feel fatigued and hungry; as your body pulls fluid from cells to dilute rising blood sugar levels, you can become crossing-the-desert thirsty as well—even though you may be sufficiently hydrated.

If not controlled, diabetes can lead to serious complications, including kidney failure, amputation, heart attack, stroke, and blindness.

Being overweight—even just a few pounds—increases your chances of getting diabetes, especially if you store fat around the waist. Of people with type 2 diabetes, 90 percent are overweight. Other risk factors include:

- Age greater than 45 years
- Gestational diabetes during a previous pregnancy
- Family history of diabetes
- Low "good" cholesterol (HDL—high-density lipoprotein—under 35 mg/DL)
- High triglycerides
- High blood pressure (140/90 or more)
- Low fitness and activity levels
- Metabolic syndrome
- Polycystic ovary syndrome

As obesity rates have gone up in the United States, so has the incidence of diabetes. At present, more than 20 million people—roughly 7 percent of the population—have the condition, but an estimated 6.2 million of them are not aware of it. If you suspect diabetes, get checked.

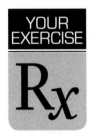

Exercise is one of the best weapons against type 2 diabetes or any problems your body has processing glucose. Regular workouts can trigger weight loss and muscle gain, both of which help your body handle glucose. But even exercise without weight loss can help: A 2013 study showed that increased exercise volume in study subjects improved blood sugar tests even when they had no change in body mass index (BMI). Also another study showed that people with diabetes cut their insulin use by $2,700 per year when they added regular activity to their lifestyle. Here are some ideas on how to improve or prevent type 2 diabetes.

STARTING IMMEDIATELY, you should incorporate as much NEAT (nonexercise activity thermogenesis) as possible into your day—meaning, get up from your chair as often as you can. Sitting in a chair for hours at a stretch causes blood sugar to spike: You're not burning any energy to speak of, so it just pools in your bloodstream, wondering what to do.

In the beginning, simply cutting down on your sitting time—by doing housework, taking get-up-and-stretch breaks from work, and short, periodic strolls throughout the day—will help enormously. Keep this up, even when you start to do more formal exercise (see "Become a NEAT Freak" on page 170).

SOME STUDIES SUGGEST that people with diabetes and prediabetes (high blood sugar) might benefit from more intense forms of exercise, above and beyond traditional aerobic exercise. One 2007 study published in the *Annals of Internal Medicine* found that an exercise program combining strength training and aerobic training was more effective at controlling blood sugar than either training method by itself.

HIGH-INTENSITY TRAINING—short periods of fast, intense exercise followed by periods of rest—has also been shown to be very effective in controlling blood sugar. One 2009 study concluded, "The efficacy of a high intensity exercise protocol, involving only about 250 kcal of work each week, to substantially improve insulin action in young sedentary subjects is remarkable."

A similar, informal case study was documented on the BBC show *Horizon* in "The Truth about Exercise." Michael Mosley, a relatively inactive doctor-cum-investigative reporter with a family history of diabetes, performed just a single minute of high-intensity stationary cycling—in three 20-second intervals, separated by 2 minutes of rest. After a month of doing three of these mini-workouts a week—12 minutes of exercise *in total*, mind you—Mosley's blood glucose improved 24 percent.

Other studies have shown that HIT-style training can be more effective at raising the aerobic capacity of people with diabetes by increasing their ability to tolerate exercise in general and improving quality of life more substantially than traditional aerobic exercise training. It may also be more effective in burning fat than traditional aerobic exercise.

HIT isn't for everyone—in order for it to work, you've got to be working near your max for those short periods. But it's very effective, and extremely time efficient. For more on how to do these types of workouts, turn to Part 3.

IF YOU ARE SEDENTARY and have weight to lose, your first step should be to simply start walking for at least a half hour a day on most days of the week, either all at once or in increments of 10 minutes or so. Improved fitness helps control the symptoms of diabetes independent of weight loss—so don't worry about the number on the scale at first; be diligent about exercise and your diabetes symptoms will improve.

KEEP A SNACK with you when you exercise—a piece of fruit or fruit juice, for example—to take in case your blood sugar drops too low.

WORK OUT WITH A PARTNER who knows you have diabetes and knows what to do when your blood sugar drops too low.

WEAR A MEDICAL IDENTIFICATION TAG or carry a card indicating you have diabetes.

EXERCISE INCREASES YOUR INSULIN SENSITIVITY and is therefore a key component of self-care for people with type 2 diabetes. Discuss your exercise options with your health care provider, however he or she may make specific recommendations.

THE PREVENTION Rx FOR TYPE 2 DIABETES: Can exercise help prevent the onset of diabetes— even in people who are at risk?

In the early 2000s, Dr. David Nathan of Harvard Medical School pioneered a study to answer that question. More than 3,200 overweight, prediabetic men and women from various ethnicities were randomly divided into four groups, which received different treatments. One group received intensive training in diet, physical activity, and behavioral modification. Their goal was to lose 7 percent of their current body weight through a combination of eating less fat, consuming fewer calories, and exercising 150 minutes a week above current levels. Other groups took medication or a placebo.

Their findings? After 3 years, researchers concluded that their lifestyle intervention measures prevented the development of diabetes in these high-risk individuals 58 percent of the time. Significantly, the tested medication was found to be only about half as effective.

A 7 percent reduction in body weight is a challenge, to be sure—but it's also a realistic, attainable goal for most people. So if you're borderline diabetic, know that your fate is very much in your hands. Motivation enough?

When to Call a Doctor

If you have any diabetic symptoms, see a doctor. Managing diabetes requires a doctor's care and supervision. In addition to lifestyle modifications, you may need medication to help regulate your blood sugar, increase your supply of insulin, or make cells more insulin sensitive.

If you or your health care provider suspects diabetes, you will probably have your blood sugar tested in a fasted state using the fasting plasma glucose test (FPG). An FPG reading of between 100 and 125 mg/dl signals prediabetes; 126 or higher signals diabetes. Another useful test measures hemoglobin A1C, or how much glucose adheres to your red blood cells, revealing how your body processes sugar over a several-month period. Any A1C reading over 5 puts you in the danger zone.

THE PROBLEM:
High Cholesterol

THE SYMPTOMS: High cholesterol is one of the more insidious problems described in this book: You can't feel its symptoms, but it's potentially very dangerous. High cholesterol is a precursor to *atherosclerosis*, a narrowing of the arteries that can cause heart disease as well as stroke, heart attack, and possibly Alzheimer's disease. It's measured by a blood test.

THE BREAKDOWN: Cholesterol isn't all bad. It's essential for proper liver and cell functioning, and for the production and functioning of hormones like testosterone and estrogen. Cholesterol isn't fat, by the way: It's a waxy, fat-like substance, 75 percent of which is manufactured in your liver. Only 25 percent comes from your diet.

In order to make its way through your bloodstream, cholesterol binds with an *apolipoprotein*, forming a passenger-transporter pair called a lipoprotein. Lipoproteins come in different types, based on how much fat they can carry: The more fat in each molecule, the less stable it is and the more health problems it can stir up.

Every 5 years or so after the age of 20, adults should have a lipoprotein profile taken, which measures the amounts of the different types of cholesterol circulating through your blood while you're in a fasted state. The test gives you a handful of basic numbers:

• **HDL (HIGH-DENSITY LIPOPROTEIN, THE "GOOD" CHOLESTEROL):** Large, heavy molecules of HDL can make up about a third of your circulating cholesterol, and are responsible for carrying excess cholesterol from your organs and other tissues back to the liver, where it's broken down and discarded. HDL is good stuff, the janitor of the circulatory system, and high HDL is a sign of good health. A good reading is about 50 mg/dl, and 65 is even better.

• **LDL (LOW-DENSITY LIPOPROTEIN, THE "BAD" CHOLESTEROL):** LDL is responsible for shuttling cholesterol from the liver to your organs and other tissues. It carries more fat and less protein, and so breaks apart more easily than HDL. Once broken down, LDL can bind with other substances and stick to your arterial walls, clogging them up. As arteries narrow over time, your heart has to work harder to circulate blood, raising blood pressure and increasing your chances of cardiac issues. For most people, an LDL reading of 100 mg/dl is healthy—but people with a risk of heart disease should aim lower.

• **IDL AND VLDL:** Intermediate-density and very low-density proteins, respectively, are even less dense than LDL, and can be equally, if not more, detrimental to the circulatory system. You probably won't get separate IDL and VLDL readings in a standard blood test, but it's worth asking your doctor for them.

• **TRIGLYCERIDES:** When you consume too many calories, too much sugar, or too much alcohol, triglycerides accumulate in the bloodstream and are eventually stored as fat. High triglycerides are a classic symptom of overeating. A reading above 150 mg/dl puts you at risk for metabolic syndrome, diabetes, obesity, and other metabolic issues.

Once you have all the numbers on each type of fat in your blood, they're combined to provide your total cholesterol (which should be less than 200) and your cholesterol ratio—the ratio between total cholesterol and HDL (which should amount to four-to-one or less).

Depending on which arteries become blocked, high cholesterol can lead to a number of different problems. Atherosclerosis—hardening of the arteries—slows bloodflow to the heart and can cause angina (chest pain), or a heart attack if a blood vessel is completely blocked. If a blood vessel leading to your brain is blocked, or bursts, you can suffer a stroke as the oxygen-deprived brain tissue becomes damaged or dies off. If vessels leading to your limbs (often the legs) are affected, you may develop peripheral vascular disease.

People with diabetes are particularly prone to high cholesterol due to the large amounts of glucose in their blood can sugarcoat circulating LDL and make it more likely to form plaque, stick to the arterial walls, and cause a blockage.

Some of the risk factors for high cholesterol are out of your control: aging, family history, and gender (older women are more likely to have high cholesterol due to a postmenopausal drop in HDL).

But even if you've been dealt a rough genetic hand, you have two important weapons: exercise and diet.

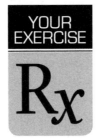

Working out boosts your HDL levels, lowers triglycerides, and may lower LDL levels as well. In a 2007 study, one hundred sedentary 50- to 75-year-old men and women were placed on an endurance training program and saw substantial improvements in blood lipid profiles: total cholesterol, triglycerides, and LDL all went down while HDL went up. This happened independent of changes in body composition—meaning that the subjects didn't have to lose weight for their numbers to improve.

A second study found that cholesterol readings for habitual exercisers were better than those of lean sedentary men—reinforcing the idea that it's exercise, and not simply being thin, that makes the difference. The study concluded that time spent on exercise was in fact the "only significant predictor" of total cholesterol and LDL levels that they could find.

And these are only two of the scores of studies that exist linking exercise to better lipid profiles. The evidence is very compelling—and in my opinion, indisputable.

For improving cholesterol readings, you don't need to go all-out: A moderate or low-intensity brisk walk works just as well as climbing Everest. And it doesn't seem to matter which type of exercise you do: Jogging, cycling, and strength training all work, and a variety of types of exercise may work even better. Yet another reason not to skip an evening stroll, even if you haven't been able to make it to the gym that day.

THE DIET PRESCRIPTION FOR CHOLESTEROL

• **UNDERSTAND HOW DIET AFFECTS CHOLESTEROL.** Few people develop high cholesterol from eating cholesterol-rich foods like eggs and lobster. The more likely dietary culprits are certain fats and carbohydrates.

• **LOWER YOUR SATURATED FAT INTAKE.** Some experts have suggested that saturated fat does no harm. I disagree: Certain saturated fats are strongly linked with high cholesterol. So if your cholesterol is high, take it easy on animal proteins, especially red meat—and if you do

eat it occasionally, you might want to shoot for a closer-to-nature type, such as grass-fed bison, which has less of the harmful fat and more of the good stuff.

• **CONSUME POLYUNSATURATED AND MONOUNSATURATED FATS.** These fats mostly come from plant and vegetable sources and are liquid at room temperature. Good sources include avocados, walnuts, olive oil, peanut oil, and corn oil. These beneficial lipids lower cholesterol and blood pressure and may decrease your chances of getting type 2 diabetes.

• **TAKE YOUR OMEGA-3 SUPPLEMENTS.** Omega-3s help lower inflammation, blood pressure, and triglycerides. These oils are found in small amounts in many foods, but are abundant in fatty fish like salmon, herring, and, to a lesser extent, tuna. Fish oil supplements—and fish!—are a good idea.

• **AVOID, AVOID, AVOID TRANS FATS!** These nasty, man-made fats are found in most store-bought baked goods and crunchy things: Check food labels, or better still, buy more things that don't have labels at all—like spinach. Trans fats not only raise your bad cholesterol, they lower the good stuff. So think twice before digging into that Twinkie.

• **WATCH YOUR SUBSTITUTIONS.** Resist the urge to replace calories lost from cutting saturated fats by eating refined carbohydrates, which can raise triglycerides and increase your chances of diabetes and obesity. An NIH study showed that people on a low-carb diet actually had better HDL levels than those on a low-fat diet. So if you're going to limit something, make it the white bread and sugary snacks.

• **EAT MORE FIBER.** Whole grains, oatmeal, and some cereals are sometimes touted as being heart healthy because the fiber in these foods can lower LDL. But be savvy about it: In recent years, food manufacturers have started dusting their worst-offender food choices with tiny amounts of fibrous dust in order to stick a "good for you" label on the box. Don't be fooled. As much as possible, I'd recommend getting your fiber from fruits, vegetables, nuts, and beans. Top off your tank with some natural whole grains like quinoa, brown rice, buckwheat, and spelt.

When to Call a Doctor

Since you won't feel your cholesterol climbing, you should have it checked at least once every 5 years—more often if you have a family history of heart disease.

THE PROBLEM: Low Thyroid (Hypothyroidism)

THE SYMPTOMS: Low thyroid hormones can make you feel tired, weak, or depressed; they can make your skin dry and your nails brittle; you may be constipated and have trouble withstanding cold or thinking clearly. Women may have irregular or heavy menstrual flow.

THE BREAKDOWN: The thyroid is a butterfly-shaped gland located in the front of the neck just below the larynx. The pituitary gland, located in the base of the brain, controls your levels of the thyroid hormones T3 and T4 through the secretion of TSH, or thyroid-stimulating hormone. In turn, thyroid keeps your metabolism running at an appropriate speed: The more thyroid you have circulating, the faster your metabolism. The higher your thyroid levels, the more energy you burn; the lower your thyroid, the less you burn. This makes it a pretty critical hormone for weight control, as well as many other functions in the body.

Thyroid also affects the way your body responds to exercise: T3 stimulates growth of new muscle and helps muscles to contract quickly during exercise. Higher levels of T3 stimulate growth of muscle tissue that is specifically responsible for speed, strength and power; lower T3 levels cause a shift toward endurance-based muscle fibers.

If you have *hyperthyroidism,* or excessive thyroid, you may experience heart palpitations, shaky muscles, and weight loss. Typically, hyperthyroidism is caused by a condition called Graves' disease, which can cause the entire gland to swell and requires medical attention.

If you have *hypothyroidism,* or low thyroid, your metabolism slows down, you're fatigued, and you gain weight. Hypothyroidism is particularly common in women going through menopause. It can be caused by a number of other conditions:

- **HASHIMOTO'S THYROIDITIS,** in which the immune system attacks and destroys the thyroid gland

- **A LACK OF IODINE** in your diet (rare in developed countries)

- **SURGERY** for hyperthyroidism

- **RADIATION TREATMENTS** for cancer

- **LOW TSH**

Both hyper- and hypothyroidism can result in reduced sensitivity to insulin, and thus, you may have a tougher time digesting high-sugar or high-carbohydrate foods such as bread, rice, and potatoes. Stress can also make low thyroid worse.

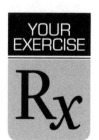

YOUR EXERCISE

The hard science is still out on the long-term effects of exercise on thyroid levels. In the short term, however, exercise definitely stimulates the thyroid gland, makes other tissues more sensitive to the effects of those hormones and increases insulin sensitivity—all good news to people with hypothyroidism.

Exercise—particularly aerobic exercise—also gives you a nice mood boost, which can be very helpful in combating the depressed mood and lethargy that sometimes comes with hypothyroidism.

Aerobic and strength training are definitely recommended, but I would also suggest interval training: short bursts of hard work followed by rest periods of equal or longer duration, which can have a powerful effect on glucose metabolism. Since they're over fast, they're a good option for people without a lot of energy to dedicate to exercise.

Try the following workout up to three times a week:

1. CHOOSE A CARDIO ACTIVITY. Virtually any activity will do, but you have to be able to work at a high intensity for at least 1 minute—so walking on a flat surface might not be challenging enough. If you're overweight, choose a low-impact activity like riding a stationary bike. Swimming does not work particularly well for this workout.

2. WARM UP FOR 5 MINUTES. Pedal, run, climb, jump rope, whatever, at an easy pace for 5 minutes. Call that a level 2 . . . on an effort level of 0 to 10.

3. GO AS HARD AS YOU CAN FOR 1 MINUTE. Try to finish a 1-minute round stronger and faster than you began it.

4. GO EASY FOR 2 MINUTES. Drop back to a level 2 effort and sustain that for 2 minutes.

5. REPEAT STEPS THREE AND FOUR according to your level of experience:

> **WEEK ONE:** Do three 3-minute rounds (9 minutes total).

> **WEEK TWO:** Do five 3-minute rounds total (15 minutes in all).

> **WEEK THREE:** Do seven 3-minute rounds total (21 minutes in all).

> **WEEK FOUR AND BEYOND:** Do six to eight rounds total, depending on your energy level.

6. COOL DOWN FOR 3 MINUTES. Drop down to an easy level 3, spin or jog for 3 minutes, and call it a day.

- Never work so hard that you can't complete all the prescribed rounds!

- If you get bored with one form of cardio, feel free to switch it up: Though they're brief, these workouts are very challenging. The key at the beginning will be learning how hard to push at each level. And feel free to move through the program at your own pace, taking even a few months' time to get up to seven or more rounds.

When to Call a Doctor

Hypothyroidism should be managed with help from your doctor. It will show up on a simple blood test, which a doctor will be likely to request if you are experiencing low-thyroid-like symptoms (which can masquerade as stress or depression as well). If other interventions don't effectively raise your thyroid levels, your health care provider may prescribe medication for the condition.

THE PROBLEM:
Metabolic Syndrome

THE SYMPTOMS: Although different health organizations offer slightly different parameters for this condition, both the National Cholesterol Education Program (NCEP) Adult Treatment Panel and the World Health Organization (WHO) agree that metabolic syndrome involves some combination of the following symptoms:

- An accumulation of belly fat
- Elevated blood pressure
- Poor HDL cholesterol panel; poor serum triglycerides
- Elevated fasting blood glucose

The two organizations offer slightly different values for each category. Both say that not all traits need to be present to be diagnosed with metabolic syndrome: The NCEP's Adult Treatment Panel states that any three justify a diagnosis; the WHO states that it *must* include elevated fasting blood glucose or post-meal glucose and any two of the other traits.

Clearly you'll need the help of a health care professional to determine if you have metabolic syndrome. But if you're overweight, sedentary, and have a family history of type 2 diabetes, hypertension, and early heart disease, you are at risk.

WHAT'S GOING ON: Metabolic syndrome, identified in the 1980s, is a cluster of metabolic disorders, all associated with an elevated risk of cardiovascular disease. It's surprisingly common, and not only among people who are overweight: About 5 percent of people of normal weight have the condition, as compared with 22 percent of people considered overweight, and 60 percent of people considered obese.

Obesity and genetics are the primary risk factors for metabolic syndrome, but other factors also increase your risk as well, including age (postmenopausal women are more likely to contract the condition), smoking, eating a high-carb diet, inactivity, and, interestingly, consuming an alcohol-*free* diet. (That's hardly a license to binge-drink, however: Just a half a drink per day is associated with the lowest risk of chronic disease.)

Metabolic syndrome is an important warning sign for conditions like type 2 diabetes, heart disease, and problems in the liver and kidney, and is also associated with a greater risk of dementia and cognitive decline in older adults.

If you have metabolic syndrome, it's largely on you to change your ways. Doctors can prescribe medication for some of your symptoms, but lifestyle changes are number one in managing this condition.

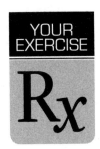

YOUR EXERCISE

Exercise, perhaps even more than diet, is your first line of defense in both preventing and treating metabolic syndrome. Due to increased risk of heart attack, however, people with this condition should be sure to follow their doctor's recommendations for exercise parameters, particularly with regard to intensity.

The American College of Sports Medicine recommends 30 to 60 minutes of moderate-intensity aerobic activity combined with at least 2 days a week of resistance training for people with metabolic syndrome. You should also try to incorporate more incidental movement throughout your day in the form of walking, housework, and other activities.

MY PRESCRIPTION: Turn to Part 3 and begin your new fitness journey. Weight loss should be your primary goal, so you should also begin to clean up your diet—see Part 4 for recommendations. Know, however, that additional activity helps reduce your chances of developing chronic disease even if you *don't* lose weight, so don't be discouraged if the number on the scale doesn't budge. Continue with your diet and exercise programs and know you're doing yourself a world of good.

When to Call a Doctor

If you have metabolic syndrome, work with your doctor on designing and implementing lifestyle changes to help you recover. He or she may also prescribe medication to help you manage high cholesterol, lipids, and high blood pressure. It's truly up to you to manage this condition, however: Your risk of sliding from metabolic syndrome into chronic disease rests almost entirely on the life choices you make, day in and day out.

THE PROBLEM:
Visceral Fat (Central Obesity)

THE SYMPTOMS: Fat accumulation around the *viscera*, or internal organs of the abdomen and trunk, that generally results in a protruding abdomen and a potbellied, apple-shaped appearance. *Visceral fat*, which lies beneath the abdominal wall, is different from *subcutaneous* fat, which lies on top of it (that's the layer you can pinch). A waist measurement of over 40 inches for men, and over 35 inches for women, or a waist-to-hip ratio of .9 or greater for men or .85 or greater for women, is indicative of visceral fat, also known as "central obesity"—fat accumulation concentrating around the abdomen.

WHAT'S GOING ON: Visceral fat isn't just bad news for your appearance. Over the last few years, research has uncovered a striking correlation between visceral fat and two major health issues: heart disease and type 2 diabetes. The more fat you've got accumulated around your middle, this research shows, the more likely you are to come down with one of these serious conditions.

What causes visceral fat? "Too much food" and "not enough exercise" are the easy answers, but smoking, insomnia, stress, and consuming estrogenic foods like beer, coffee, and soy may also contribute to the problem.

Men with the classic, firm "beer belly" have visceral fat. Though some women develop visceral fat, their "problem areas" are typically in the lower body. And though it drives some women to distraction come bathing-suit season, accumulated fat on your legs and hips is actually *cardioprotective*—meaning it's associated with a *lower* incidence of heart disease.

If you've got a lot of noticeable fat gathering around your waist, however, take it seriously.

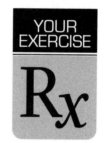

YOUR EXERCISE

Losing weight can seem like an overwhelming task, particularly if you're carrying a lot of extra weight. When your target weight is 30, 50, 100 or more pounds away, the temptation can be to give up very quickly if you don't see big changes from the outset.

Medically speaking, though, the most significant benefits of exercise come when you go from doing *nothing* to doing *something*. So if you're completely sedentary, know that just adding a half-hour walk a few times a week will make a substantial difference in your health. And if you manage to lose the first few pounds— say, 10 or 15—your health markers improve measurably as well. So even if your target weight remains many months, pounds, and workouts away, know that your exercise habit is still doing your health a world of good.

Some guidelines:

• Vigorous, large-muscle group activity, three times a week; more mild structured activity 2 additional days a week, less sitting, and increased activity overall.

• A better diet: there's no way around it for visceral fat—you've got to improve your diet. Turn to Part 4 for some smart, practical tips on eating for fat loss.

• Although some studies show a *slight* tendency for the body to burn fat in areas adjacent to working muscles, *spot reduction*—burning fat from specific areas of the body—is largely a myth.

• Lots of work on the core muscles will not burn off visceral fat. Although exercise of any type and duration will *help,* studies are showing that the more you do, and the harder you work at it, the better luck you'll have.

Why higher intensity? A 2011 study published in *Medicine & Science in Sports & Exercise* found that high-intensity exercise—performed at about 75 to 80 percent of maximum aerobic capacity—is much more effective in burning abdominal fat than a lower-intensity program (50 to 60 percent of max) of the same duration.

When to Call a Doctor

Obese people should consult with their doctor—and possibly a trainer—to come up with a workable plan to help them burn off the extra baggage. If an underlying problem—such as a thyroid condition—is present, a medical professional will oversee your treatment for that as well. Your doctor may suggest specific activities to avoid (high-impact activities may be out due to the stress they may cause your lower body), and others to do more of (walking, cycling, and strength training often work well for people with lots of weight to lose) as you embark on your exercise program.

CHAPTER 4

Hormonal and Sexual Problems

What activity gets your heart pumping, reduces stress, lifts your spirits, and improves your relationships?

If you said "exercise," you'd be right. And if you said "sex," you'd be right, too. Exercise can be a rising tide that improves everything, including sexual and hormonal functioning (which leads to rising temperatures, heart rates, and, um, body parts—all good!). This is true for both genders. Some of it is physical. Improved circulation can aid erectile dysfunction, for example, and aerobic exercise can alleviate some of the cardiovascular changes that occur with menopause. But improvements can also be psychological: Sexual functioning can be a reflection of how you feel about yourself and your body. And as you'll soon discover, if you haven't already, exercise improves that, too.

THE PROBLEM:
Erectile Dysfunction (ED)

THE SYMPTOMS: Difficulty achieving and maintaining an erection. Lots of men *occasionally* have this problem—and it often causes far more concern and embarrassment than it's worth, because one-off erectile problems are attributable to any number of factors, including stress and fatigue. True ED is a chronic condition and deserves your attention—not only for the sake of your sex life, but because it may signal more serious health problems.

WHAT'S GOING ON: For most guys, a penis is like a car: They don't worry about how it works until it doesn't. And when that happens, life stops.

Getting and maintaining an erection is a fairly complex mechanical process: During sexual arousal, the brain sends chemical messages to the nerves in the penis to relax contracted blood vessels, allowing blood to flow freely into *corpora cavernosa*, the two parallel, cylindrical chambers of spongy tissue that make up the bulk of the penis. High pressure traps this blood inside the penis, and *voilà*—he's standing at attention.

Despite what you may have heard, ED is not always "all in your

head." There are many possible causes for ED, and a lot of them are physical:

- Cardiovascular problems like heart disease

- Neural conditions like Alzheimer's, Parkinson's, multiple sclerosis, and stroke

- Metabolic problems like obesity and diabetes

- Smoking and alcohol

- Antidepressants and other prescription drugs

- Radiation therapy

- Surgery of the bladder and lower digestive tract

- Psychological causes like stress, performance anxiety, and depression

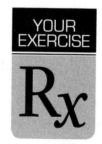

YOUR EXERCISE Rx

Great news: Erectile dysfunction is very responsive to exercise. Regular workouts directly combat many of the causes of ED, including stress, poor sleep, and problems with circulation, self-image, and self-esteem. Exercise also helps fight obesity, and may make it possible to go off antidepressants—though you must see your doctor before altering your dosage.

Any type of lower-body exercise—running, brisk walking, hiking, and, especially calisthenics and lower-body strength training—may be particularly effective in helping to alleviate symptoms of ED because of their effect on circulation below the waist. The one exception to this is long-distance cycling and mountain biking, particularly on bikes with long, narrow seats. Such seats can put undue pressure on the perineum—the area between the anus and the scrotum—and obstruct circulation through an artery that supplies blood to the penis. Recent studies, published in the *Journal of Sexual Medicine,* have indicated that even "ergonomic" seats can cause these problems. If you're a serious cyclist, take a break every 45 minutes during long rides. And if you experience numbness during cycling, or develop ED symptoms, take a break from cycling—or at the very least, get yourself a new seat.

All told, however, with the possible exception of stopping smoking, exercising is by far the best step you can take for an ongoing and satisfying sex life.

When to Call a Doctor

If erectile dysfunction is chronic and does not respond to smoking cessation and regular exercise, mention it to your doctor (don't be embarrassed—it's what we're here for!).

ED can be an early harbinger of cardiovascular disease, since a good erection is all about good bloodflow. If your circulatory system is becoming unhealthy, the smaller blood vessels—like in the penis—could be the first ones affected. Having an exam may be the smartest thing you ever do.

It's also possible your doctor may test for low testosterone, which can also cause ED. Depending on the results of that test, you might be put on hormone replacement therapy as well.

Some guys, however, simply want a fast cure to a disturbing problem. You might be tempted to go the easy route and hit up a doctor for an ED pill like Viagra before you've tried exercising. And given how commonplace such prescriptions are, your doc might acquiesce. But don't you think you'd feel better if you got your mojo back on your own?

THE PROBLEM:
Health Changes Due to Menopause

THE SYMPTOMS: Menopause often has unpleasant side effects, including weight gain, hot flashes, urinary incontinence, sleep disruptions, pain during sex and loss of sex drive, and other physical changes.

WHAT'S GOING ON: Just one woman in four gets through menopause without major symptoms. Half experience moderate symptoms, and 25 percent have more severe symptoms. It's not an easy time.

At birth, females have 1 to 3 million eggs. Throughout a woman's life, these eggs slowly die off—some through ovulation, but most through a natural process called atresia—until, at menopause, a woman may only have about 10,000 eggs. Around this time, these eggs become more resistant to the reproductive hormone FSH (follicle-stimulating hormone), which stimulates growth, and the ovaries reduce their production of estrogen.

Because estrogen plays a vital role in maintaining the health of the blood vessels, heart, uterus, breasts, skin, bone, and brain, loss of the hormone is considered the cause of many of the symptoms of menopause, including weight gain (espe-

cially around the middle) and increased chances of cardiovascular disease, osteoporosis, obesity, and other chronic diseases. Testosterone production also drops off in women around this time, often resulting in a decline in libido.

Hormone therapy—taking estrogen and other hormones in pill, gel, or cream form—can alleviate hot flashes, but also has been shown to carry significant risks of heart disease, stroke, blood clots, and breast cancer. For most women, therefore, this type of treatment is probably not worth the risk.

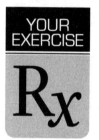

YOUR EXERCISE

Although menopause is a natural consequence of reaching middle age, many of its undesirable side effects are avoidable. A 2006 study found that middle-aged women who started an exercise program saw a marked reduction in symptoms after 12 months; in a control group of women who had no exercise at all, symptoms got worse.

In a 2004 review of previous studies, researchers at the UKK Institute for Health Promotion Research found that aerobic exercise improved health markers in postmenopausal women, including bone-mineral density, body weight, body-fat percentage, blood pressure, and metabolic fitness.

Finally, in a 2012 study of postmenopausal women, exercise was shown to influence a little-known health marker: *telomere length*. Telomeres are the endcaps on I-shaped chromosomes, resembling the caps on the ends of shoelaces, which protect the cells from long-term deterioration. Short telomeres are associated with many age-related health issues, among them cardiovascular disease, stroke, cancer, diabetes, declining cognitive function, and arthritis. By contrast, younger and healthier people have longer telomeres.

Unlike some age-related changes, shortening of the telomeres can be slowed, and even reversed, with lifestyle choices like smart exercise habits.

For some great ideas, see "The Best Exercises for Menopause" on the next page.

When to Call a Doctor

See a doctor for moderate to severe symptoms, or if you experience symptoms before age 45. Women who experience menopause early have a higher risk of osteoporosis, coronary heart disease, depression, anxiety, Parkinson's, and changes in sexual function, and might be better candidates than older women for hormone therapy.

THE BEST EXERCISES FOR MENOPAUSE

In studies, postmeno-pausal women who saw the most benefits from exercise worked out a full 60 minutes a day, 4 days a week or more, doing a combination of aerobic and strength work. That should be a goal.

In addition to strength work, women 50 or older should focus on developing power— the ability to move quickly. Not only will that improve coordination and prevent falls, it also helps maintain bone density, counteracting the bone loss that also accompanies menopause. The best way to do this is with plyometrics— fast jumps performed with full power in sets of 5 to 10.

Finally, I also recommend yoga, tai chi, Pilates, or other internal, mind-body practices for stress and anxiety a few times a week.

LOWER-BODY, QUADRICEPS EMPHASIS (3 SETS OF 12)
STRENGTH TRAINING: Perform three times a week, choosing at least one move from each of the following categories every workout.

BODY-WEIGHT SQUAT
Place your fingers on the back of your head and pull your elbows back so that they're in line with your body. Squat until your thighs are parallel to the floor. Hold for a second, then return to the starting position.

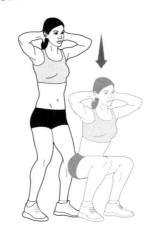

LUNGE
• Stand tall with your arms hanging at your sides. Step forward with your right leg and lower your body until your right knee is bent at least 90 degrees. Hold for a second. Return to the starting position.

• Complete the prescribed number of reps, then lunge with your left leg.

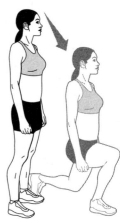

REVERSE LUNGE
• Stand tall with your arms hanging at your sides. Brace your core and hold it that way.

• Lunge back with your left leg, lowering your body until your right knee is bent at least 90 degrees. Hold for a second and return to the starting position.

• Complete the prescribed number of reps and repeat with the opposite leg.

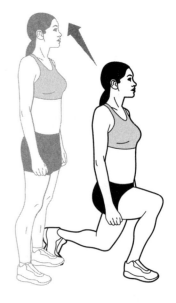

LOWER-BODY, HAMSTRING/GLUTE EMPHASIS (3 SETS OF 12)

DUMBBELL DEADLIFT

• Set a pair of dumbbells on the floor in front of you. Bend at your hips and knees and grab the dumbbells with an overhand grip.

• Without allowing your lower back to round, stand up with the dumbbells. Lower the dumbbells to the floor.

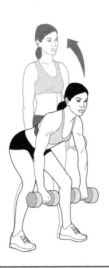

STIFF-LEG DUMBBELL DEADLIFT

• Grab a pair of dumbbells with an overhand grip and hold them at arm's length in front of your thighs. Stand with your feet hip-width apart and your knees slightly bent.

• Without changing the bend in your knees, bend at your hips and lower your torso until it's almost parallel to the floor. Pause, then raise your torso back to the starting position.

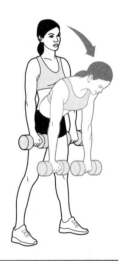

SWISS BALL HIP RAISE AND LEG CURL

• Lie faceup on the floor and place your lower legs and heels on a Swiss ball. Place your arms out to your sides at a 45-degree angle to your torso, palms facing down.

• Push your hips up so that your body forms a straight line from your shoulders to your knees.

• Without pausing, pull your heels toward you and roll the ball as close as possible to your butt. Pause for a second, then reverse the motion by rolling the ball back until your body is in a straight line.

• Lower your hips back to the floor.

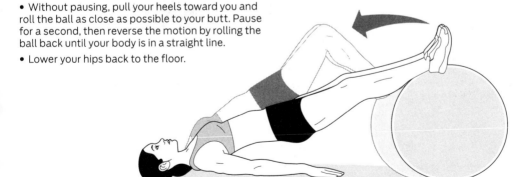

(continued)

THE BEST EXERCISES FOR MENOPAUSE—*CONT.*

PLYOMETRICS

Perform 3 sets of 10 of *one* of these exercises 3 times a week—after a warmup but before other exercise. Perform each rep at full power, taking a moment between repetitions if necessary. Focus on landing without wobbling or the knees collapsing inward.

TUCK JUMP

Stand with your feet shoulder-width apart. Dip your knees in preparation to leap. Explosively jump as high as you can. Lift your legs up into your midsection so you can grab your knees (the "tuck"). Release your knees so you land normally.

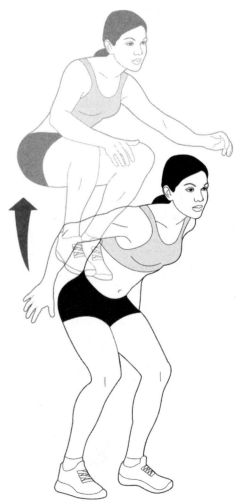

STEP-UP

Stand in front of a bench or step and place your right foot firmly on the step. Press your heel into the step and push your body up until your right leg is straight. Pause for a second, then lower your body back down until your left foot touches the floor, then repeat. Halfway through the time allotted, switch feet.

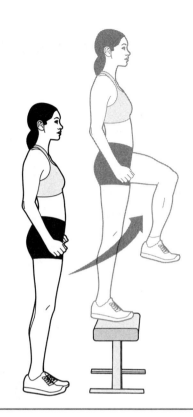

SKATER JUMP

Stand on your right foot with your right knee slightly bent and place your left foot just behind your right ankle. Bend your right knee and lower your body into a partial squat. Then bound to the left by jumping off your right foot. Land on your left foot and bring your right foot behind your left as you reach toward the floor with your right hand. Repeat the move back toward the right, landing on your right foot and left hand. The entire motion mimics a speed skater.

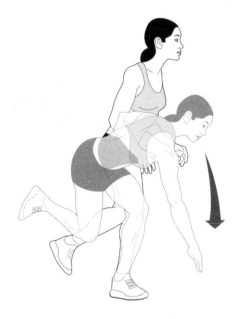

THE BEST EXERCISES FOR MENOPAUSE—*CONT.*

UPPER BODY, PUSH (3 SETS OF 10)

PUSHUP

• Get down on all fours and place your hands on the floor so that they're slightly wider than and in line with your shoulders. Your body should form a straight line from your ankles to your head.

• Lower your body until your chest nearly touches the floor. Pause at the bottom and then push yourself back to the starting position as quickly as possible. If your hips sag at any point during the exercise, your form has broken down.

NOTE: If necessary, perform "modified" pushups, following the same instructions, but with your knees on the ground.

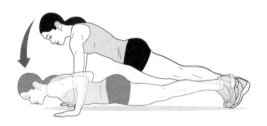

DUMBBELL BENCH PRESS

• Grab a pair of dumbbells and lie on your back on a flat bench, holding the dumbbells over your chest so that they're nearly touching.

• Lower the dumbbells to the sides of your chest. Pause, then press the weights back up to the starting position as quickly as you can. Straighten your arms completely at the top of each repetition.

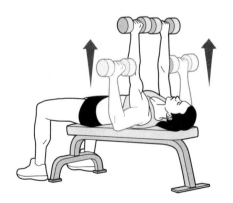

DUMBBELL SHOULDER PRESS

• Stand holding a pair of dumbbells just outside your shoulders with your arms bent and palms facing each other. Set your feet shoulder-width apart, knees slightly bent. Brace your core.

• Press the weights upward until your arms are completely straight. Slowly lower the dumbbells back to the starting position.

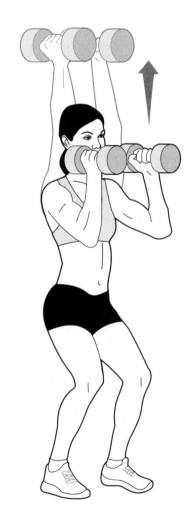

UPPER BODY, PULL (3 SETS OF 10)

INVERTED ROW

• Lie on the floor beneath a stationary bar. Grab the bar with an overhand, shoulder-width grip. Your body should form a straight line from your ankles to your head.

• Initiate the movement by pulling your shoulder blades back, then continue the pull with your arms to lift your chest to the bar. Pause, then slowly lower your body back to the starting position.

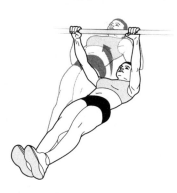

LAT PULLDOWN

• Sit down in a lat pulldown station and grab the bar with an overhand grip that's just beyond shoulder width. Your arms should be straight.

• Without moving your torso, pull the bar down to your chest as you squeeze your shoulder blades. Don't lean back. Pause, then slowly return to the starting position.

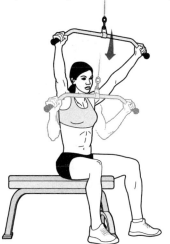

CHINUP

• Grab the chinup bar with a shoulder-width, underhand grip. Hang at arm's length. Cross your ankles behind you. You should return to this position—known as a dead hang—each time you lower your body back down.

• Pull your chest to the bar. Once the top of your chest touches the bar, pause, then lower your body back to a dead hang.

NOTE: If traditional chinups are too challenging, per-form negative chinups: Set a bench under a chinup bar, step up on the bench, and grasp the bar using a shoulder-width, underhand grip. From the bench, jump up so that your chest is next to your hands, then cross your ankles behind you. Try to take 5 seconds to lower your body until your arms are straight. Jump up to the starting position and repeat.

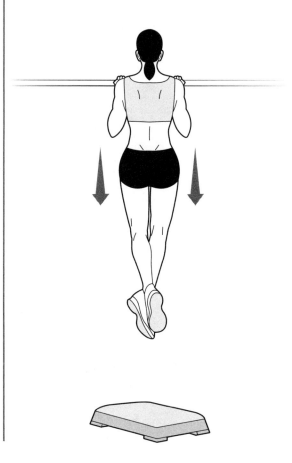

THE PROBLEM:
PMS
(Premenstrual
Syndrome)

THE SYMPTOMS: In women of childbearing years, physical and emotional disturbances occur during the luteal phase—after ovulation and before menstruation—of the menstrual cycle, including

- Tension
- Bloating
- Breast tenderness
- Food cravings
- Crying spells
- Headaches and backaches
- Fatigue
- Irritability
- Anxiety
- Weight gain
- Severe cramping
- Trouble concentrating

People joke about PMS—but there's no doubt it can be rough, even in mild cases. And if you have severe, recurrent PMS, it can bring on its own form of misery for many days out of the month.

WHAT'S GOING ON: Clinically speaking, a diagnosis of PMS is only given when the symptoms are primarily emotional, rather than physical, and are severe enough to interfere with some aspects of your life—work, relationships, family, or other obligations. Only about 2 to 10 percent of women experience this degree and type of PMS. By a looser definition, however, as many as 85 percent of women of childbearing years experience premenstrual symptoms that range from mild to severe.

PMS is caused by hormonal shifts that accompany the menstrual cycle. Fluctuating levels of the neurotransmitters serotonin and beta-endorphin, both of which play a role in mood regulation, may also be a factor.

You can't cure the symptoms of PMS completely, but you can certainly manage and contain their severity.

Common remedies include:

- **NSAIDS** (nonsteroidal anti-inflammatory drugs) like Advil, which can help lessen severe cramping

- **A BALANCED DIET** that includes plenty of fiber

- **REGULATION OF SUGAR** and caffeine intake

- **ADEQUATE SLEEP** and rest

- **ORAL CONTRACEPTIVES.** This can be very effective in regulating periods and easing the physical symptoms of PMS, though this treatment typically does not address emotional symptoms.

- **IN STUBBORN CASES, SSRIS** (selective serotonin reuptake inhibitors), a class of antidepressants, can be effective in easing emotional symptoms

And you need to include regular exercise. See below.

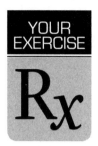

If you've got intense PMS symptoms, including cramps, anxiety and depression, and mood swings, you may feel inclined to get in bed and stay there. Resist the urge: Movement will help with hormonal shifts, keep menstrual flow going, and reduce cramps. Unless you're given specific instructions from a doctor, there's no reason to stop exercising at any phase of your menstrual cycle.

A UK review of multiple studies confirmed—in each study—that all subjects who exercised reported a reduction in PMS symptoms. To relieve these symptoms, the following ideas may be particularly helpful:

- **GO AEROBIC.** Plenty of anecdotal evidence, and some studies, have suggested that aerobic exercise is helpful in reducing mild PMS symptoms—possibly more so than strength training. Being consistent about aerobic exercise during the last 10 days of your cycle may be more important than exercising long or hard. Check the workouts in Part 3 for some good ideas.

- **TAKE A YOGA CLASS.** In a 2012 study, 61-points relaxation, a yoga-style workout, proved effective in lowering stress in premenstrual women. The tension-relieving stretches and deep breathing associated with yoga workouts may help relieve both the physical and emotional effects of PMS. See "Five Yoga Stretches for PMS" on the following pages.

When to Call a Doctor

Most cases of PMS can be self-managed, but if PMS is severe and inhibits you from performing daily activities, call a doctor. In conjunction with smart lifestyle adjustments, a number of prescription drugs can also help ease your symptoms.

FIVE YOGA STRETCHES FOR PMS

One useful note when you're premenstrual (and if you're new to yoga): Avoid a lot of twisting moves, inversions, and poses that activate your abdominal muscles. The moves that follow are terrific for PMS symptoms.

1. CAT POSE (BIDALASANA)

Assume an all-fours position. Keeping your arms straight, slowly arch your back so that your belly and chest go toward the floor, your shoulder blades come together, and your head lifts toward the ceiling. Breathe deeply and hold for 30 seconds, attempting to sink more deeply into the pose each time you exhale.

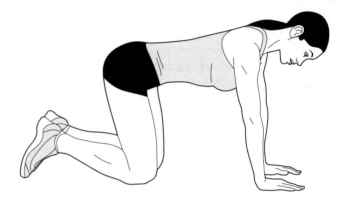

2. BOW POSE (DHANURASANA)

Lie on your belly. Bend both knees so that your heels come toward your butt. Reach back, grab your ankles, and slowly arch your back, lifting your head and legs and squeezing your shoulder blades together. Breathe deeply and hold for 30 seconds.

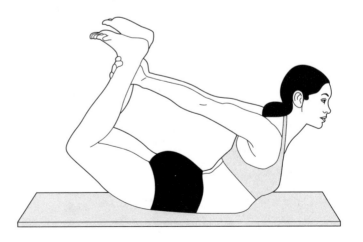

3. COBRA POSE (*BHUJANGASANA*)

Lie on your belly and place your hands on the floor beneath your shoulders as if you are about to perform a pushup. Keeping your hips on the floor, press your torso upward, look forward, and squeeze your shoulder blades together. Breathe deeply and hold for 30 seconds.

4. FISH POSE (*MATSYASANA*)

Lie on your back with your legs straight and together, toes pointed, arms by your sides. Slowly press your elbows into the floor, lift your chest as high as possible, and squeeze your shoulder blades together, allowing your head to tilt backward. Breathe deeply and hold for 30 seconds, attempting to lift your chest slightly higher each time you exhale.

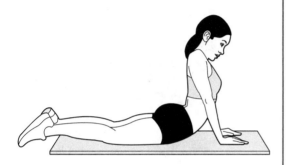

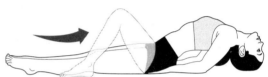

5. CORPSE POSE (*SAVASANA*)

Lie on your back with your legs a comfortable distance apart, arms on the floor. Relax completely into the floor and breathe easily.

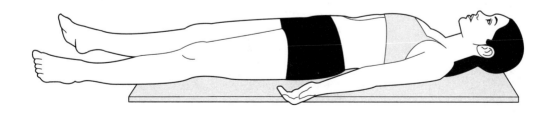

THE PROBLEM:
Low Libido

THE SYMPTOMS: A significant, sustained drop in your own desire or performance, an uncharacteristic lack of enthusiasm for sex in yourself or your partner, or simply a new rash of resentment and negative feelings surrounding sex.

WHAT'S GOING ON: In *Annie Hall*, Woody Allen and Diane Keaton are discussing their sex life together, in split screen, with their respective therapists. Asked how often they have sex, Allen tells his therapist, "Hardly ever! Three times a week!" Responding to the same question, Keaton replies, "Constantly. Three times a week!"

What constitutes a satisfying sex life, or a stagnant one, is highly subjective. And over a long relationship, sex can become a higher or lower priority because of kids, job pressure, hormonal changes, and other life stressors. Illness of all kinds can cause a loss of sex drive, from minor health problems like a cold to more serious health problems like thyroid disease and tumors of the pituitary gland. Low testosterone may also result in a stagnation of sexual activity for men. Certain antidepressants, blood pressure medications like Clonidine and Methyldopa, and the anti-psychotic drug chlorpromazine can also affect libido.

In a committed relationship, many factors affect sexual activity and response. Fatigue and stress are among the two most common causes—especially financial stress: According to a 1992 study, women in a household where income fell 20 percent were 1.5 times more likely to report low desire as those where income remained stable; men in such households were more likely to experience erectile problems.

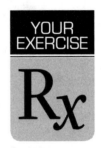
YOUR EXERCISE

Exercise addresses many of the direct causes of low libido. A 2004 study of college students, published in the *Electronic Journal of Human Sexuality*, found a strong correlation between fitness levels and self-reported feelings of desirability in both men and women. In men, frequency of exercise was also related to positive feelings about sexual performance. Since the quality of your sex life often reflects your feelings about *yourself* as much as it does your feelings toward your partner, these findings are significant.

Another reason for regular exercise for better sex: The fitter you are, the better your overall sexual performance will be. Losing weight, building strength, and increasing flexibility will allow you to be more physically capable of exciting, fun, and satisfying sex.

The type of exercise is less important here than the plan: couples workouts. Exercising with your partner may be one of the best and most fun ways to bring some spark back into your sex life. It's a twofer: Not only can you bond and motivate each other, you get to watch your partner get physical. Cycling, jogging, or hitting the gym together can set the stage for getting sweaty together in private later in the day. And what's dancing, of course, if not a socially acceptable form of public foreplay?

When to Call a Doctor

Most problems with a stalled sex life can be addressed through open communication with your partner and taking the usual measures to protect your health, including exercise. If your sex life has taken an uncharacteristic nosedive, however, and none of the other common factors are present (unusual stress or fatigue, lack of exercise, illness, relationship stress), then you should consult a doctor. Although it's rare, occasionally an unusually low libido may be the only detectable cause of a more serious, underlying health problem.

THE PROBLEM:
Low Testosterone

THE SYMPTOMS: In men, erectile problems and infertility; low energy, decreased mental acuity, and aggressiveness; lower strength and stamina; loss of bone density and greater susceptibility to injury. Weight gain, high blood pressure, and other cardiovascular conditions may also result. In men and women, a drop in sex drive and performance. Low testosterone, or *hypogonadism*, in men is defined as anything below 350 nanograms per deciliter of testosterone, detectable in a simple blood test.

WHAT'S GOING ON: Like you learned in sex-ed class, testosterone is the hormone that makes a man look and sound like a man. When a boy hits 13 or 14, a puberty-driven testosterone spike causes his voice to deepen, his muscles to thicken, his penis and gonads to grow. Women, too, secrete testosterone via the ovaries and the adrenal glands, although at a rate of only about 1/20th of the amount present in men. In adulthood, testosterone is responsible for the maintenance of a large number of functions, including energy levels, fertility, sex drive, muscle and bone growth, and a general sense of well-being.

In men, testosterone generally hits a high-water mark around age 20 and declines at a rate of about 1 percent a year starting around age 40,

sometimes dropping to the point where men feel they are experiencing a significant hormonal shift, or "male menopause." Other conditions or events can also cause a precipitous drop-off in testosterone levels, however, including:

- Injury to the testicles
- Testicular cancer and its treatments
- HIV/AIDS
- Chronic liver or kidney disease
- Obesity
- Type 2 diabetes
- Chronic stress

Testosterone levels also fluctuate in response to various everyday activities as well: Watching your favorite sports team prevail in a major contest may cause it to spike, for example, whereas cuddling or playing with children can cause it to dip.

Although many men believe that more testosterone is inherently beneficial, and even seek hormonal treatments to "top off their tank," it isn't always true. Men with exceptionally high testosterone—1,000 nanograms or more—are more likely to commit crimes, or drink and smoke to excess. They also tend to get injured, lose their jobs, and engage in any number of risky and irresponsible behaviors more frequently than men with levels closer to normal.

Most men seem to function best when testosterone levels are at a moderate level of approximately 400 to 600 nanograms.

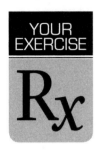

• **LIFT HEAVY THINGS:** Numerous studies have shown a link between increased testosterone and exercise, particularly strength training. If you think your testosterone may be low, choose large-muscle-group exercises like squats, deadlifts, and power cleans. Use plenty of weight—85 percent or more of what you can handle for a single repetition, or, alternatively, use less weight but perform a high volume of exercise, 4 to 6 sets of 5 to 8 reps per exercise. Avoid a lot of long, slow cardiovascular exercise like jogging.

• **REST AND RECOUP:** Too *much* exercise, on the other hand, can also lower your "T" levels. So don't exercise the same muscle groups 2 days in a row, rest at least a minute between sets, and keep your sessions down to two or three a week per muscle group. If you're an endurance athlete, limit your long runs or bike rides to once a week, and focus on short-to-medium efforts the rest of the time.

• **DE-STRESS:** Elevated cortisol, which commonly results from stress, can lower testosterone levels. Keep stress at bay by going to sleep at a reasonable hour, taking short breaks throughout your workday, and eating healthy meals.

When to Call a Doctor

Many of the initial symptoms of low testosterone are vague, such as fatigue, listlessness, and nonspecific aches and pains. Others, like erectile problems, are more obvious (though ED may have other causes as well). If you are experiencing difficulty achieving and maintaining an erection, your doctor will in all likelihood check your levels. Low testosterone is not serious, and is treatable with medication if exercise and other nonmedical interventions prove ineffective. A simple blood test is all you need, and you should get results back in 1 or 2 days.

CHAPTER 5

Musculoskeletal Problems

My years in sports medicine have led me to believe that the standard directive for pain and injury—rest, ice, compression, and elevation, or RICE—needs some amending. Every injury has its own treatment needs, but in general, I feel that "total rest" when you have a muscular or skeletal injury is bad advice.

In most cases of back pain, for example, I suggest moving as soon as possible: Get up off the couch and bear crawl or crab walk around the house if necessary, but get yourself moving. In the case of other injuries, stay away from painful movements and perform rehab according to your doctor's suggestions—but go hard on movements that don't irritate the injury. Getting creative with new and different activities might even improve your health and fitness!

Exercise is too powerful and effective a medicine to lay off just because some part of you is temporarily sidelined. Bloodflow will increase, even to the injured area, your spirits will lift, and you'll remind yourself that you're strong enough to overcome setbacks of all kinds. This section will show you the smartest ways to get yourself back out there—and back on the road to being 100 percent as quickly as possible.

THE PROBLEM:
Poor Flexibility

THE SYMPTOMS: Your joints feel tight and creaky; your muscles and connective tissue feel wound tight; twisting or bending your spine in any direction may feel challenging or unpleasant. This isn't an injury, per se, but it's a physical issue that could lead to injury—and it definitely holds you back in any activity.

WHAT'S GOING ON: To work properly, all muscles need to be able to both contract and extend. For example, bend your arm and your biceps contract while your triceps extend. Straighten your arm and the triceps contract while the biceps extend. This ability of a muscle to extend comfortably over its full range is its *flexibility*.

If the muscle is short, or tense, your full range will be limited. Ditto if the *fascia*, a tough tissue that wraps around and interweaves through the muscles, or the tendons, which attach the muscles to your bones, are short or tight. Injury, inactivity, poor posture, poorly coordinated movement, and genetics—how flexible your parents are—can directly affect the length of these tissues.

Tension in your muscles is another big factor that affects flexibility. Most muscles have some degree of tension—or *tonus*—in them all the time, even when you feel as if you're relaxed. Muscle tension can be affected by injury, stress, heavy work, or hard exercise, and by repetitive movements with a small range of motion.

How much tension you hold, and where you hold it, is an individual matter: Some people habitually carry more tension in their muscles than others. There are loosey-goosey folks who don't seem to have a bone—much less a tight muscle—in their bodies; conversely, there are those who are more bound up. One 2004 study found that athletes in different sports—and even different positions within the same sport—showed different patterns of flexibility and tension throughout their bodies.

Over time, tight muscles can become more than a minor inconvenience: One inflexible muscle group can eventually cause muscle groups on the opposite side of a joint to stop working altogether. As that muscle group sits on the sideline, still other muscles have to step in and pick up the slack. This domino effect can eventually cause even the most basic movement pattern—like walking or driving—to become uncoordinated and painful.

When the hip flexor muscle group on the fronts of your hips becomes short, for example—a common consequence of sitting—the front of your pelvis gets pulled forward and down when you stand. Your lower back then has to work extra hard to pull you upright, and the biggest muscles in your body— your butt muscles—suddenly have a hard time doing their job. A host of problems can result: back pain, tight hamstrings, a rounded back, a head that protrudes forward, painful shoulders. Eventually, other problems related to poor movement—including sciatica—can develop. A similar cascade of problems can occur when the flexibility limitation occurs in the upper back and neck.

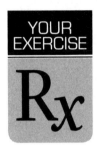

Clearly, all of us need *some* amount of flexibility training to avoid pain and to move comfortably through our everyday life. The real question: *How much and what kind of flexibility training does the average person need?*

The key with flexibility is not how far you can stretch, but to keep all your moving parts in a more or less balanced relationship, so that nothing is either too tight *or* too loose.

There are three stretching modalities I particularly like: *foam rolling* and *dynamic stretching*, which you should do before any workout, and *yoga*, which you can do afterward. Foam rolling is huge. I love it. For the full rundown on how to do it, go to page 180.

In dynamic stretching, you're essentially practicing athletic movement—and I'm a big proponent of all things athletic. In yoga, you're learning to relax and be comfortable in fully extended, stretched positions. All of these can be workouts in their own right.

And here's a bonus prescription: You'll also find "The Desk-Sitter's Flexibility Secrets" in the following pages as well. These are static stretches (meaning you're not moving a body part, you're holding a stretch) that are crucial for people who spend a lot of time sitting in front of a screen. All that sitting can destroy your posture, which leads to all sorts of lousy outcomes from lower back pain to inhibited breathing (try breathing deeply while you're hunched over, as opposed to sitting with your back straight and shoulders back). These stretches, though not tied to any workout or warmup, should be done throughout any day when you're sitting a lot.

You can do all of these types of stretches anywhere and anytime. As long as you're not injured, you almost can't do them enough. But stick with foam rolling and dynamic stretches before a workout—they'll help you perform with optimal speed and strength—and yoga-like stretches afterward, which will help you cool down and unwind. Yoga stretches are also terrific first thing in the morning and before you go to bed.

When to Call a Doctor

Some autoimmune conditions, such as rheumatoid arthritis and fibromyalgia, can cause stiffness and inflexibility in the joints, particularly following sleep or after a prolonged period of sitting down. You could also have an overuse injury, a bone disease, or cancer. Feeling stiff for more than 30 minutes after getting up and moving around, or having an unexplained, sudden loss of flexibility, generally or in one specific area, may be a warning sign of osteoarthritis or another more serious condition. Call a doctor and get it checked.

DYNAMIC STRETCHING

These anywhere, anytime stretches are a terrific way to increase flexibility for everyday activities and sports alike. Use them as a warmup before a workout or as a quick energy booster at any time throughout your day. Also, check out the foam rolling section on page 180.

DIRECTIONS:
Move into each stretch at a deliberate speed, hold for a one count, then come out of it slowly. Repeat each stretch 8 to 10 times per side.

WALKING HIGH KNEES
Stand tall with your feet shoulder-width apart. Without changing your posture, raise your left knee as high as you can and step forward. Repeat with your right leg. Continue to alternate back and forth.

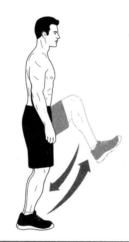

LUNGE WITH SIDE BEND
• Stand tall with your arms hanging at your sides. Step forward with your right leg and lower your body until your right knee is bent at least 90 degrees.

• As you lunge, reach over your head with your left arm as you bend your torso to your right. Reach for the floor with your right hand. Return to the starting position.

• Complete the prescribed number of reps, then lunge with your left leg and bend to your left for the same number of reps.

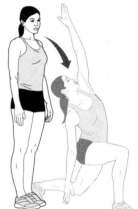

FLOOR Y-T-I RAISES
NOTE: Do 8 to 10 reps of each.

Y RAISE
Lie facedown on the floor. Allow your arms to rest on the floor, completely straight and at a 30-degree angle to your body, your palms facing each other (thumbs up). Your body should resemble the letter Y. Raise your arms as high as you can, pause, then slowly lower back to the starting position.

T RAISE
Lie facedown on the floor. Move your arms so they're out to your sides—perpendicular to your body with the thumb sides of your hands pointing up—and raise them as high as you can. Pause, then slowly lower back to the starting position.

I RAISE
Lie facedown on the floor. Position your arms straight above your shoulders so your body forms a straight line from your feet to your fingertips. Your palms should be facing each other, thumbs pointing up. Raise your arms as high as you can, pause, then slowly lower back to the starting position.

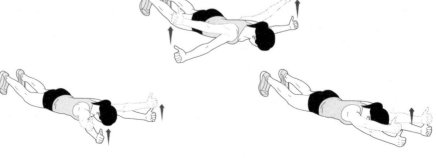

REVERSE LUNGE WITH REACH BACK

• Stand tall with your arms hanging at your sides. Brace your core and hold it that way. Lunge back with your right leg, lowering your body until your left knee is bent at least 90 degrees.

• As you lunge, reach back over your shoulders and to the left. Reverse the movement back to the starting position.

• Complete the prescribed number of reps with your right leg, then step back with your left leg and reach over your right shoulder for the same number of reps. Keep your torso upright for the entire movement.

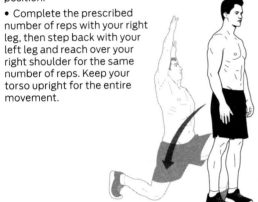

LOW SIDE-TO-SIDE LUNGE

• Stand with your feet set about twice shoulder-length apart, your feet facing straight ahead. Clasp your hands in front of your chest (dumbbells optional).

• Shift your weight over to your right leg as you push your hips backward and lower your body by dropping your hips and bending your knees. Your lower right leg should remain nearly perpendicular to the floor. Your left foot should remain flat on the floor.

• Without raising yourself back up to a standing position, reverse the movement to the left. Alternate back and forth.

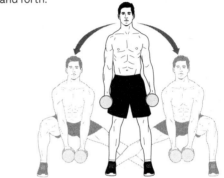

INCHWORM

• Stand tall with your legs straight and bend over and touch the floor. Keeping your legs straight, walk your hands forward. (If you can't reach the floor with your legs straight, bend your knees just enough so you can. As your flexibility improves, try to straighten them a little more.) Keeping your core braced, walk your hands out as far as you can without allowing your hips to sag.

• Then take tiny steps to walk your feet back to your hands. That's one repetition. Do 5 forward, and then 5 more in reverse.

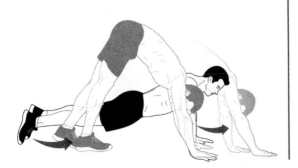

INVERTED HAMSTRING

• Stand on your right leg, your knee bent slightly. Raise your left foot slightly off the floor. Without changing the bend in your right knee, bend at your hips and lower your torso until it's parallel to the floor.

• As you bend over, raise your arms straight out from your sides until they're in line with your torso, your palms facing down. Your left leg should stay in line with your body as you lower your torso.

• Return to the start. Complete the prescribed number of repetitions on your right leg, then do the same number on your left.

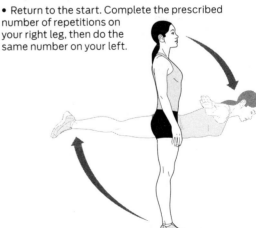

FIVE EVERYDAY YOGA STRETCHES

Yoga isn't just for the latte-sipping crowd anymore. This ancient practice is great for stress and pain reduction as well as building athleticism and flexibility. Try this brief routine after a workout or as a way of de-stressing and focusing your energy during the day.

For best results, hold each *asana,* or pose, for 30 seconds to 1 minute, breathing deeply and slowly through your nose. Breathing is key. If you are unable to perform the pose as described without undue discomfort, back off a bit (reaching for your shins rather than the feet on the forward bend, for example, or placing a small block or bench underneath your hands on the camel pose).

Although *asanas* appear to be static, they are actually very active: As you breathe, you will probably find yourself able to deepen into each stretch.

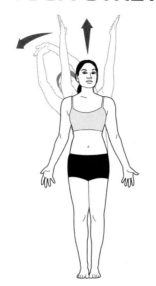

1. MOUNTAIN

Stand with your feet together and big toes touching. Relax your shoulders and lengthen your neck. Let your arms relax along your sides, palms to the front, and gaze forward. Optional: Raise your arms straight above your head, palms facing in, elbows facing out. Add in a side stretch by leaning to one side, then repeating for the other side.

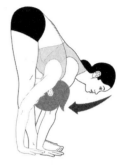

2. FORWARD BEND

Stand with your feet together, arms at your sides. Exhale as you bend forward at your hips, reaching your hands toward the floor. Imagine folding your body in half.

NOTE: For beginners, bend as far as you can and hold for 30 seconds, making sure to breathe slowly and deeply.

3. DEEP LUNGE

Stand with your feet shoulder-width apart. Step forward with your right leg and lower yourself until your right leg is bent 90 degrees and your left knee is almost touching the ground. Keep your weight resting on the heel of your front foot and the ball of your rear foot. Raise your arms straight up over your head, keeping them shoulder-width apart. Keeping your arms straight, bring your palms together. Hold for 30 seconds, return to the starting position, and repeat for the left leg.

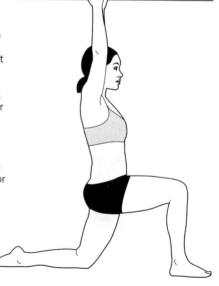

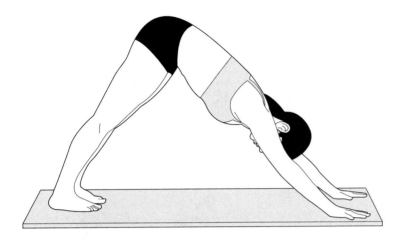

4. DOWNWARD-FACING DOG

Begin on all fours with your knees hip-width apart and your hands shoulder-width apart. Your hips should be over your knees and your shoulders over your wrists. Walk your hands a few inches in front of your shoulders. Curl your toes under, lift your hips, and straighten your legs. Push into your palms to draw more energy into your lower body to help elevate your pelvis. Keep your arms straight and have your body form an upside-down V.

5. TRIANGLE

Stand with your feet one leg-length apart. Rotate your left foot out to a 90-degree angle and your right foot inward to a 45-degree angle, keeping your heels aligned. Lift your arms out to your sides until they're parallel to the floor. Bend to your left and extend your left arm to the floor outside your left ankle. Your right arm should point to the sky, and your right shoulder should be vertical with your left. Keep your core engaged and your legs straight. Hold for the specified time, then switch to the opposite side.

THE DESK-SITTER'S FLEXIBILITY SECRETS

Different people have different flexibility needs. But the majority of people these days need stretches that will *undo* the tightness and tension that result from lots of sitting. Here, you'll find seven anywhere-anytime stretches you can do—maybe on a break from work—that will help to keep you from slumping into a permanently chair-shaped posture. Hold each one for 30 seconds.

HIP FLEXOR STRETCH WITH OVERHEAD REACH

• Assume a lunging position with your right foot forward, your left knee on the floor, and both knees at a 90-degree angle. Extend your right arm overhead.

• Keeping your torso upright, your hips and shoulders square, and your left knee on the floor, step your right foot forward about 12 inches and push your hips forward and downward until you feel a deep stretch in the front of your left hip. Hold for 30 seconds and repeat on the other side.

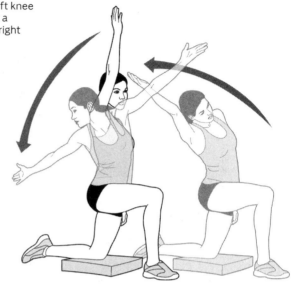

DOORWAY CHEST STRETCH

• Bend your right arm 90 degrees (the "high-five" position) and place your forearm against a door frame. Stand in a staggered stance, your right foot in front of your left.

• Rotate your chest to your left until you feel a comfortable stretch in your chest and the front of your shoulder. Hold for 30 seconds. Switch arms and legs and repeat for your other side. Repeat for a total of 3 reps on each side.

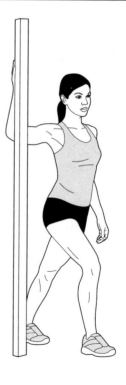

WALL CALF STRETCH

• Stand about 2 feet in front of a wall in a staggered stance, your right foot in front of your left. Place your hands on the wall and lean against it.

• Shift your weight to your back foot until you feel a stretch in your calf. Hold this stretch for 30 seconds on each side, then repeat twice for a total of 3 sets. Perform this routine daily, and up to 3 times a day if you're really tight.

LYING SPINAL TWIST

• Lie on your back with your arms directly out to your sides, palms up, your knees bent, and your feet flat on the floor.

• While keeping your feet together, simultaneously lower your knees toward the left and roll your head toward the right. Hold for 30 seconds and repeat on the other side.

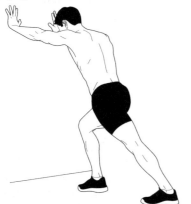

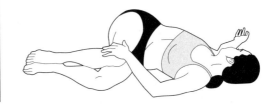

KNEELING QUADRICEPS/HIP FLEXOR STRETCH, BACK LEG UP AGAINST THE WALL

• Assume a lunging position with your left foot forward, your right knee on the floor, and both knees at a 90-degree angle. Extend your right arm overhead. Keeping your torso upright, your hips and shoulders square, and your right knee on the floor, step your left foot forward about 12 inches and push your hips forward and downward until you feel a deep stretch in the front of your right hip. Hold for 30 seconds and repeat on the other side.

• Place a gym mat next to a wall. Face away from the wall and assume a kneeling lunge position on the pad with your left knee down and your right foot flat on the floor in front of you. Slide backward toward the wall, pointing the toes of your left foot toward the ceiling. Keeping your left knee on the floor, inch your foot up the wall behind you until you feel a comfortable stretch in the front of the left thigh. Place both hands on your right knee and extend your back into an upright posture. Hold for 30 seconds and repeat on the other side.

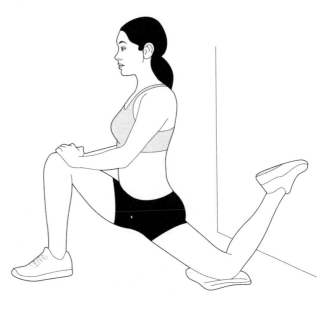

THE PROBLEM:
Muscle Strain

THE SYMPTOMS: Pain, and possibly swelling, bruising, or even a complete rupture in a muscle, usually following overuse; sudden, unexpected contraction; or trauma. Also known as a "pull" or a "tear."

WHAT'S GOING ON: A strain is a tear in a muscle group that can also affect the tendon that attaches the muscle group to the bone. Strains are graded on a scale of one to three.

• **GRADE ONE** involves a tearing of up to 10 percent of the fibers in a muscle. You may experience a twinge and pain for 2 to 5 days afterward, but you can function fairly normally.

• **GRADE TWO** tears up to 90 percent of the fibers in a muscle. You may experience swelling or bruising, and most movements that involve the area will be very painful.

• **GRADE THREE** tears more than 90 percent of the muscle fibers, including a complete rupture of the muscle. You'll need immediate medical attention and, depending on the affected area, possibly surgery as well.

Mild muscle strains are very common: Just work an area a little bit too hard—in the weight room, on the track, or moving the couch in your living room—and you can strain something. Indeed, it's tough to go through

life—active or sedentary—without straining a muscle now and then.

Often strains occur when you've violated the "rule of toos," and done "too much, too soon, too fast." Before a good warmup, muscle tissue resembles a bungee cord on a cold morning: stiff, unable to stretch easily, and is therefore much more susceptible to injury than later in the workout. On the other hand, strains also occur in the heat of athletic competition, when adrenaline is pumping and you decide to go for that desperation move to score a goal or stop an opponent. Heck, you can strain a muscle *sneezing*.

The point? You never quite know when strains will happen. But you can take steps to prevent them. When they do happen, you can hasten their recovery while maintaining your overall fitness. Finally, once the area has healed, you can strengthen and mobilize it to make sure you don't strain the area again.

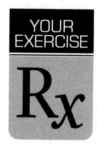

YOUR EXERCISE

You don't want to exercise a strained muscle: It needs rest and time to knit back together. Instead, you should employ the dynamic rest technique I previously mention on page 19.

MOVEMENT: Of everything, that is, that doesn't affect the injured area. Full rest is bad medical advice: You'll lose fitness, your circulation and healing will slow, and your mental outlook can turn negative. So work around the pain: If your injury is in your upper body, like a pectoral strain, perform lower-body workouts. If it's a calf strain, stick with swimming, upper-body strength training, and cycling, if you can do it without pain. But don't let the injury sideline you completely: Keep moving as much as possible, and if that movement is limited, raise the intensity of your activity to maintain or increase your fitness.

ICE: Ice the injured area 4 to 6 times a day for 15 minutes for the first 2 days. You can also take NSAIDs (nonsteroidal anti-inflammatory drugs like ibuprofen).

COMPRESSION: Depending on the location and type of strain, you can wrap it with a compression bandage to help bring the torn ends of the muscle closer together so they can heal more easily. Never compress a nerve compression injury, however.

ELEVATION: Raise the affected area above the level of your heart to reduce inflammation.

Once you're past the stage where moving the area hurts (which could take anywhere from a few days to a few months, depending on the severity of the tear), you'll want to rehab it. A sports doctor or physical therapist will have specific instructions for this. In general, however:

1. EASE INTO STRETCHING: Gently stretch and mobilize the area through a pain-free range up to several times a day. You'll increase circulation and rebuild the mobility you'll need to get back to full activity.

2. WORK IT—GENTLY: At first, depending on the severity of your strain, you may not be able to contract or lengthen a muscle under pressure. In that case, you can try isometric contractions: contracting a muscle without moving it. For example, for a strained pectoral muscle hold the top position of a pushup, with your arms just slightly bent.

• **FROM THERE,** you can move onto eccentric contractions: slowly lowering a weight under some kind of load. If you've strained your quadriceps, you might do an eccentric lunge or squat.

• **NEXT,** you can work the injured muscle concentrically—meaning, contracting the muscle while it's loaded: doing one-legged heel raises for a strained calf, for example. If you still have pain, work any concentric movement slowly, so as not to reinjure the area.

• **FINALLY,** you can get back to full activity—gradually. That would involve faster, more explosive movements: sprinting, explosive pushups, and the like, which put a lot of stress on muscles.

CAUTION: Some people strain muscles because they're not used to explosive or fast movement. Make sure that once you're back up to speed, you gradually include some faster, more explosive moves in your training program so you're ready to exert this kind of force when the situation demands it.

When to Call a Doctor

If walking or other normal functions are painful or difficult, and if relief doesn't come from basic home treatment like icing and taking anti-inflammatories like ibuprofen or naproxen, see a doctor. An MRI can determine the extent of the damage to your muscle or tendon, and the doctor may prescribe more specific stretching, strengthening, or physical therapy exercises. In very rare cases—a full rupture—surgery may be recommended.

THE PROBLEM:
Muscle Weakness

THE SYMPTOMS: Lack of ability to contract some or all of your muscles with normal force.

WHAT'S GOING ON: The most common reason that people become weak in the long term is inactivity: Just as muscles grow and get stronger when you exercise, they shrink and get weaker when you don't. Age-related sarcopenia, or muscle atrophy, is a common condition in older adults—though whether aging or simple inactivity is to blame is not altogether clear.

Short-term muscle weakness is quite common as well. Usually, it happens when you're tired or overworked and your body can't provide enough energy to fuel additional muscle contractions. If you've ever run all-out for any period of time, or done a long, tough set of lunges, you know what I'm talking about: it's the "Jell-O legs" feeling that you get when you've pushed yourself to your absolute limit.

Here's the deal: All movement in your body is ultimately powered by *adenosine triphosphate,* a supercharged molecule that stores the energy we need to function. Some ATP is stored right in your muscles, but most of it is made to order, using one of these two basic mechanisms:

- *AEROBIC* **PATHWAY,** in which the body uses fats and oxygen, and

- *ANAEROBIC* **PATHWAY,** in which the body uses glycogen, a form of sugar stored in the muscles.

Most of the time, you run on the aerobic system, which works great—provided you're not working too hard. Push yourself a little harder, however, and your aerobic system can't keep up with the demands you're putting on it. In that case, the *anaerobic* metabolism kicks in to provide you with some fast fuel.

Trouble is that the anaerobic metabolism is only good for about 90 seconds of all-out effort before it gets temporarily depleted. At the same time, burning all that sugar produces by-products—hydrogen ions, mostly—which start to accumulate in your muscles, slowing down muscle contraction, making the muscles ache, and giving you those telltale Jell-O legs—a condition known as *peripheral fatigue.* Certain types of hard exercise can also bring on DOMS, or delayed-onset muscle soreness, tenderness and pain in the muscles, which can sometimes last several days.

Another reason you might get temporarily weak is due to *neural fatigue:* Your nervous system can't generate the sustained, high-frequency signal your muscles need to contract in the way you want them to. In that case, you might not feel much discomfort in your muscles at all, because the problem isn't there. It's in the nerves that are trying to get the signal through to your muscles.

Finally, you can have *central fatigue,* a temporary, systemic condition in which your body seems unable to generate significant force—you just feel weak as a kitten. Central fatigue is probably a protective mechanism, which kicks in when too much force may cause damage to vital organs, such as when you're sick or seriously sleep-deprived.

Some more serious medical conditions may also cause muscle weakness, including Addison's disease, thyroid issues, multiple sclerosis, a pinched nerve, stroke, or a spinal issue. Generally speaking, weakness of this kind comes on suddenly in one specific area and is not related to activity or exercise.

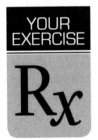

Assuming you're cleared for activity and don't have a serious medical condition (see "When to Call a Doctor"), the fastest and best way to get stronger is through strength training. Strength training has numerous benefits for people experiencing muscle weakness: Very quickly, it affects neural efficiency, which improves your capacity to generate strength. After a few weeks, it causes muscle fibers to *hypertrophy,* or grow in size. It increases movement speed and

strength and your ability to generate anaerobic—sprint-type—speed and power.

If anything, strength training is more essential for older adults than for younger people. As we age, we lose type-II muscle fibers (those responsible for fast or strenuous movement), while type-I muscle fibers, those responsible for easier, longer-duration exercise, are left more or less intact. This is part of why adults who may still be able to walk long distances nonetheless may start to have trouble getting out of a chair, swatting a fly, or catching themselves when they fall: Their type-II muscle fibers have shrunk.

Use it, so the saying goes, or lose it. You can't grow or develop strength or power in muscles unless you *use* that strength and power.

Older adults, even those up to 96 years old in one study, can improve muscular strength—as well as gait speed, stair-climbing power, balance, and overall spontaneous activity—from just 8 weeks on a strength-training program.

Strength training doesn't have to be complicated: You don't need a lot of equipment—or a lot of time. Try the "Conquer Weakness" Workout on the next page twice a week. If you're sedentary now and want to dive into strength training, it's a great place to start.

When to Call a Doctor

Contact a doctor if you experience sudden, unexplained weakness, especially localized weakness not accompanied by other symptoms like a fever, or if it comes on following a viral infection. You could be experiencing one of the more serious medical conditions previously mentioned. And even if you're not, a doctor visit will be able to rule those out and identify the real problem.

THE "CONQUER WEAKNESS" WORKOUT

If you're feeling like you may have lost a step lately—or two, or thirty—don't despair: Studies have shown that resistance training can make men or women stronger at *any* age.

For your first 2 weeks, do this program twice a week on nonconsecutive days (Mondays and Thursdays, say). On week 3, do 3 sets of each move. After week 4, you can choose from a variety of workouts at the back of this book.

DIRECTIONS: Do 15 reps of each move below, rest for 1 minute, repeat, and move on to the next exercise. If it gets easy, accelerate through your reps— meaning, squat like you're trying to jump off the floor and do pushups as if you're trying to launch yourself into the air on each rep. The key: *Always* maintain proper form and lower yourself under control.

PUSHUP

• Get into pushup position, using your hands as a base.

• Keeping your body straight from your head to your ankles, lower your body until your chest nearly touches the ground. Pause at the bottom and then push yourself back to the starting position as quickly as possible.

EASIER VERSION: Hands-elevated pushups. To make the exercise easier, place your hands on a bench or on a raised sturdy object.

TOUGHER VERSION: Feet-elevated pushups. To make the exercise more challenging, place your feet on a bench or other sturdy object.

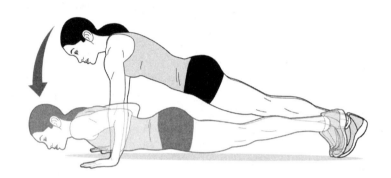

BODY-WEIGHT SQUAT

• Place your fingers on the back of your head and pull your elbows back so that they're in line with your body.

• Perform a body-weight squat until your thighs are parallel to the floor, hold for a second, then rise back up to the standing position.

EASIER VERSION: Partial squats. Follow the directions, but only lower yourself until your thighs are at a 45-degree angle to the floor.

HARDER VERSION: Jump squats. Perform a body-weight squat until your thighs are parallel to the floor, then explosively jump as high as you can (imagine you're pushing the floor away from you as you leap). When you land, immediately squat and jump again.

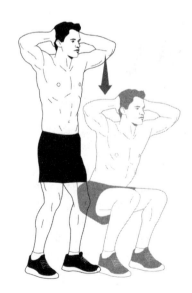

COBRA

- Lie facedown on the floor with your legs straight and your arms next to your sides, palms down.

- Contract your glutes and the muscles of your lower back and raise your head, chest, arms, and legs off the floor.

- Simultaneously rotate your arms so that your thumbs point toward the ceiling. At this time, your hips should be the only parts of your body touching the floor. Hold for a second, then return to the starting position.

EASIER VERSION: Superman. Instead of having your hands at your sides, extend them out in front of you, so when you raise your body, you resemble Superman flying.

HARDER VERSION: "Hold" cobras. Same move as above, only hold the extended overhead position for a three count.

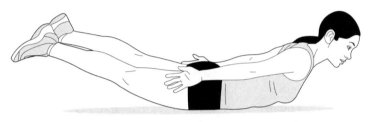

LUNGE

- Stand tall with your arms hanging at your sides.

- Step forward with your right leg and lower your body until your right knee is bent at least 90 degrees. Your left knee should not touch the floor. Hold for a second. Return to the starting position.

- Complete the prescribed number of reps, then lunge with your left leg.

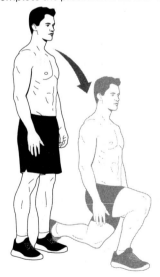

EASIER VERSION: Front-foot elevated split squat. Land your front foot on a raised area such as a step or workout box, 6 to 12 inches high.

HARDER VERSION: Rear-foot elevated split squat. Place your back foot on a raised area such as a step or workout box, 6 to 12 inches high, and keep it there as you perform your reps.

THE PROBLEM:
Performance Plateaus

THE SYMPTOMS: You're working out regularly but no longer seeing any strength or fitness gains.

WHAT'S GOING ON: The bioscience model of exercise goes something like this: train, rest, eat, improve. Repeat till death.

Reality is a little different. Everyone progresses quickly at the beginning of an exercise program, but after a few months changes come much more slowly, if at all. Your performance may hit a plateau, lasting weeks or months, during which you may be training just as hard but getting little for your efforts.

Under optimal circumstances, the body responds to training in three phases:

1. THE "SHOCK AND ALARM" PHASE, which may last days or several weeks, during which the exerciser feels very sore and can't perform up to normal standards

2. THE "RESISTANCE" PHASE, during which the body adapts to the new stimulus and returns to normal functioning

3. THE "SUPERCOMPENSATION" PHASE, during which the body builds new muscle and connective tissue, your neurons learn to fire

better, you get more coordinated, and, in general, you get better at your chosen activity

If you stress your body too much, though, and don't rest enough—or if you continue putting the same demands on your body over weeks and months—you'll reach the "exhaustion" phase, in which training may feel monotonous and become ineffective. During this phase, life stresses stemming from work, poor diet, insufficient sleep, and other issues may interfere with training progress.

Overspecialization—too much focus on a single activity—is one major cause of performance plateaus. When I was in high school, many kids did three different sports throughout the year. These days, I see many kids who are year-round soccer or baseball players: That means their bodies are absorbing the same kind of punishment, year after year, with no break. A plateau—sometimes a long one—is almost inevitable.

Everybody plateaus at some point, however, from the best-trained pro athlete to the weekend Ultimate Frisbee player. The body isn't a machine, it doesn't improve on a schedule: There are always fits and starts. Most people mistake the first plateau they encounter—or the second, or the fourth, or the tenth—for the best they can do. And that's a mistake. Because a performance plateau, most commonly, is not a signal from your body to give up, but just a gentle request to do things a little differently.

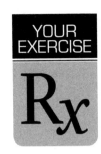

Besides patience, the solution to a performance plateau is almost always a combination of training *variety* and rest.

• **IF YOUR PROGRESS HAS STALLED,** try doing less of what you're good at and more of what you're not so great at. If you like jogging, focus on speed; sprinters may get faster by improving endurance.

Similarly, strength athletes who always focus on heavy sets of 1 or 2 reps can improve by lightening their loads a bit and doing more reps; higher-rep junkies can get a boost from training heavier.

The lesson? Do something different.

• **CROSS-TRAINING** isn't just for triathletes. When the season changes, take a break from your chosen activity and try something new. Either get away from the sport entirely, focusing on a different activity, or choose some aspect of your game you want to improve: more power on your strokes if you're a tennis player; more kick in your final sprint if you're a marathoner. Then focus on improving those qualities *generally* in the off-season, working on explosive lifting or hill sprints for several weeks. You'll come back to your actual activity fresher

and with more enthusiasm than if you just kept up a competitive-season training schedule.

• **FOR WEIGHT-LOSS PLATEAUS,** understand that calorie restriction slows down your metabolism—so early success in weight-loss efforts is bound to level off. Rather than restricting calories even further, try switching up your exercise program: Strength training, in particular, helps preserve and grow muscle mass, which keeps your metabolism humming, even as you lose fat.

• **TRUE "OVERTRAINING SYNDROME,"** in which your performance plateaus or worsens for many months, is extremely rare. Doing too much now and then, however, also called "overreaching," is quite common. The solution to an overreach? Drop your volume of training by half or more for up to a week (jump back in only when you feel fresh and excited about training again). In all likelihood, you'll come back much stronger after this backing-off period because your body will be *supercompensating* after all your hard training: growing new muscle, repairing connective tissue, building new neural pathways. Smart trainers actually include periods of deliberate overreaching into their athletes' schedules—an extra-long training day, a long run, a brutal week of training—to create this same effect. But it only works if you rest afterward!

When to Call a Doctor

Performance plateaus aren't medical emergencies. More likely you'll just want to get in touch with a good trainer or coach.

THE PROBLEM:
Ligament Sprain

THE SYMPTOMS: Pain and sometimes swelling and instability around a joint, caused by sudden twisting or bending, usually following a fall or some type of impact.

WHAT'S GOING ON: A sprain is an injury to a ligament—the fibrous tissue that connects one bone to another. Like muscle strains, they are graded in severity from one to three, one being a minor tear of 10 percent or less of the ligament, two being a partial tear of 90 percent or less, and three being a complete, or near-complete, rupture of the ligament.

Since several ligaments span each joint, sprains often affect more than one ligament at a time. They can occur in any joint, but some common ones I see include:

• **ANKLE SPRAINS,** which usually occur when your foot rolls outward (and occasionally inward) while walking or exercising on an uneven surface

• **KNEE SPRAINS,** most common when you pivot quickly while playing sports

• **WRIST SPRAINS,** which typically happen when you land on an out-stretched hand during a fall

• **THUMB SPRAINS,** which usually happen when something you're holding—commonly a ski pole or tennis racquet—torques the joint

Several factors can contribute to sprain:

POOR CONDITIONING: Weak or uncoordinated muscles don't support your joints as effectively as strong ones, which can put extra pressure on your ligaments and make them susceptible to injury.

FATIGUE: Even strong athletes get tired. Fatigued muscles behave like weak ones: They don't do their job as well as when they're fresh, so they don't support the joints as well.

IMPROPER WARMUP: Warming up changes the viscosity of muscles and connective tissue, making them more supple and bendable. It also increases your proprioception—your ability to sense your position in space—so you're less likely to take a bad or awkward step during your first few minutes of play.

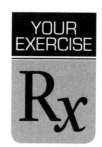

YOUR EXERCISE

Sprain a ligament or two and the old-school approach was to rest completely till it healed. As with muscle strains, I think it's better to be as proactive as possible: Play around the pain rather than letting it hobble you completely. That means *dynamic rest.*

You don't want to aggravate a sprain: Ligaments have limited blood supply and tend to heal slowly, so more stress can make the injury worse, or at least slow the healing process. So stay active while avoiding anything that causes pain or feels unstable. For mild knee and ankle sprains, try cycling instead of running; for more intense lower-body sprains, stay away from lower-body work altogether and stick with upper-body and core work in the weight room, and swimming for cardio.

With upper-body sprains, it's the same deal in reverse: If the injury is mild, you might be able to slip in some swimming, pushups, and chin-ups; if it's worse, skip all such activities, including golf, tennis, and heavy bench presses. Stick to lower-body and core work for strength and fitness instead. Never do anything that irritates the injured area. The key: Up your intensity so you maintain or improve your cardiovascular fitness.

For the first couple of days after a sprain, ice the area 4 to 6 times a day for 15 minutes at a stretch; you can also take an over-the-counter nonsteroidal anti-inflammatory drug like ibuprofen to relieve swelling and pain.

When to Call a Doctor

As a rule, I recommend a doctor visit for any kind of joint pain. Even if the injury is mild, professional evaluation can determine how badly (or not) you've hurt yourself. Most grade one (mild) sprains won't feel bad enough to warrant a trip to the doctor, and in all likelihood they'll heal on their own. But I still recommend an exam.

Grade two or three sprains will more or less drive you to the doc automatically: Normal function will be difficult or impossible.

Once there, a doctor will probably order an MRI or some other type of imaging to see the extent of the damage. In the event of a full rupture, you could need surgery—though even that depends on the type of injury.

If your sprain is severe, or it requires surgery, a doctor or physical therapist will probably suggest some at-home treatment options to stretch and strengthen the injured area. In addition to those, and in less severe cases, you can resume normal activity slowly, starting with milder types of exercise like uphill walking or pool running (if your sprain is in the lower body) or swimming or using a rowing machine if it's in your upper body. Resume more vigorous activity gradually, and stop immediately if you feel pain in the injured area.

THE PROBLEM:
Lower-Back Pain

THE SYMPTOMS: Minor to intense and debilitating pain in the lower spine, sometimes with a specific, traumatic cause, such as an injury; other times without apparent cause. The thick muscles on either side of the spine (*erector spinae*) may go into spasm; you may also experience a stabbing pain on one or both sides of the lower back. Pain can recur, sometimes coming and going over weeks and months.

WHAT'S GOING ON: Chances are you won't get through life without at least some lower-back pain: It affects from 70 to 80 percent of people in industrialized countries at some point. What causes it? Sometimes it's quite obvious: You decided you really didn't need help moving that couch, or you played that extra set of tennis. You strain something.

Very often, though, lower-back pain stems from "motor control error," which sounds like just what it is: Command-central in your brain, responsible for telling your body which muscles to turn off and which to turn on throughout your day, pulls the wrong switch while you're doing something innocuous like tying your shoes, and whammo! You're lying on your back, finding religion.

Finally, lower-back pain can be nonspecific in origin: You're

depressed, you're stressed out at work, your spouse serves you divorce papers, your teenage son gets a nose ring. Suddenly you're reaching for the Advil. You might not make the connection, but these things can cause back pain, too.

The best way to treat lower-back pain is to avoid it altogether, since people who have had lower-back pain often get it again. The best way to do that? The right kind of exercise.

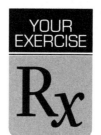

YOUR EXERCISE

Unless your doctor tells you otherwise, the last thing you should do for lower-back pain is rest: Even if movement is minimal and awkward, do your best to stay active throughout the day and throughout your recovery.

For prevention of lower-back pain *and* rehabilitation after an injury, the back-and-core-building program shown on page 116 is a great insurance policy.

In addition, observe the following guidelines, adapted from the work of Dr. Stuart McGill, professor of spine biomechanics at the University of Waterloo:

1. Perform lower-back exercises *daily.*

2. Do not exercise to the point of pain or discomfort: less pain, *more* gain.

3. Cardiovascular training—even of low intensity—is an important part of lower-back rehabilitation. Stay within the parameters recommended for healthy individuals, but avoid movements that exacerbate or bring on the pain. Lower-impact choices like swimming and cycling may be preferable to running or hiking.

4. Do not perform heavy lifting movements within an hour of waking, as high fluid levels in the intervertebral discs following sleep make them more prone to injury.

5. Use less resistance and a higher number of repetitions (15 or more) when performing exercises for the lower back and core. Endurance in these muscles appears to be more protective than strength.

6. Do not overstretch an injured lower back! Flexibility is not an essential component of recovery, and in fact, extra stretching may slow recovery or lead to reinjury.

When to Call a Doctor

Most cases of lower-back pain do not require medical attention. If yours is especially debilitating, your doctor will want to rule out possible underlying issues like osteoarthritis and spinal stenosis, and possibly prescribe muscle relaxers, which can alleviate spasms so you can begin rehab.

Disc herniation, which sounds frightening, may or may not be the cause of back pain: 30 to 40 percent of people without back-pain symptoms have herniations, while as many as 50 percent of people with back pain have no apparent herniations.

TRAIN AWAY LOWER-BACK PAIN

The most important exercise you can do for your lower back is to get up out of your chair as often as you can: Sitting weakens the muscles that surround your spine and leaves you vulnerable to injury.

During formal workouts, though, the following movements have a proven track record for being safe and effective.

FOAM ROLLING

If you've never foam-rolled before, be prepared. It's uncomfortable, and can even be painful when you start. Don't worry—the more painful it is, the more that muscle needs foam rolling. The good news is that the more you do it, the less discomfort you'll feel. For each muscle that you work, slowly move the roller back and forth over it for 30 seconds. If you hit a really tender spot, pause on it for 5 to 10 seconds.

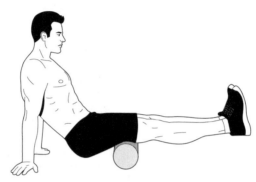

HAMSTRING ROLL

• Place a foam roller under your right knee, with your leg straight.

• Cross your left leg over your right ankle. Put your hands flat on the floor for support. Keep your back naturally arched.

• Roll your body forward until the roller reaches your glutes. Then roll back and forth. Repeat with the roller under your left thigh.

NOTE: If rolling one leg is too difficult, perform the movement with both legs on the roller.

GLUTE ROLL

• Sit with a foam roller positioned on the back of your right thigh, just below your glutes. Cross your right leg over the front of your left thigh.

• Put your hands flat on the floor for support.

• Roll your body forward until the roller reaches your lower back. Then roll back and forth. Repeat with the roller under your left glute.

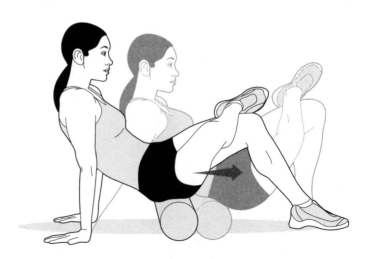

ILIOTIBIAL-BAND ROLL

• Lie on your right side and place your right hip on a foam roller. Put your right forearm on the floor for support. Cross your left leg over your right and place your left foot flat on the floor.

• Roll your body forward until the roller reaches your knee. Then roll back and forth. Lie on your left side and repeat with the roller under your left hip. (If this becomes too easy over time, place your left leg on top of your right instead of bracing it on the floor.)

IMPORTANT NOTE:
Your iliotibial band—commonly called the IT band—is a tough strip of connective tissue that runs down the side of your thigh, starting on your hip bone and connecting just below your knee. When you start foam rolling, you'll probably find that this tissue is one of the most sensitive areas that you can roll over, perhaps due to the high tension of the band. Remember, pain means you need to roll it. Make this a priority, because over time, if your IT band is too tight, it could cause knee pain.

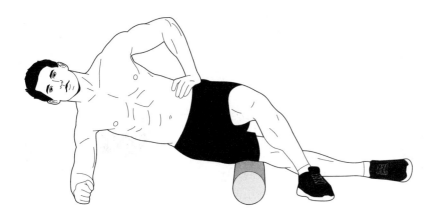

WHERE DID ALL THE CRUNCHES GO?

Ten or fifteen years ago, no lower-back-pain prevention program would have felt complete without bunches of crunches—that on-your-back half-situp move that fitness experts were telling us was the safer alternative to the full version, and the best way to isolate and build the abdominal muscles.

Well, they—or maybe I should say we—were wrong. Recently, in large part thanks to the work of spine biomechanics expert Dr. Stuart McGill, crunches have been shown to be detrimental to spine health. According to McGill, there may be no quicker way to herniate a disk than to flex the spine

forward over and over again, as in the crunch exercise.

Crunches are also what might be called a "nonfunctional" exercise. Think about it: When you're standing, walking, and otherwise going about your life, your spine is elongated, a position that the abdominal muscles help support. The only time the abs shorten into a crunch-like position is when you're getting up off the floor or slumping on the couch—not something you need any more practice doing.

I much prefer planks to crunches, as you'll see in this plan. Planks are no-impact, and you can do them anywhere.

TRAIN AWAY LOWER-BACK PAIN—*Continued*

QUADRICEPS-AND-HIP-FLEXOR ROLL

• Lie facedown on the floor with a foam roller positioned above your right knee. Cross your left leg over your right ankle and place your elbows on the floor for support.

• Roll your body backward until the roller reaches the top of your right thigh. Then roll back and forth. Repeat with the roller under your left thigh. (If that's too hard, perform the movement with both thighs on the roller.)

PLANK

• Get into pushup position, but bend your elbows and rest your weight on your forearms. Your body should form a straight line from your shoulders to your ankles.

• Brace your core and hold for 30 seconds.

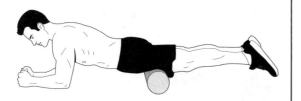

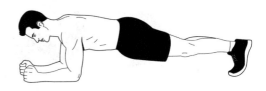

LOWER-BACK ROLL

• Lie faceup with a foam roller under your midback. Cross your arms over your chest. Your knees should be bent, with your feet flat on the floor.

• Raise your hips off the floor slightly. Roll back and forth over your lower back.

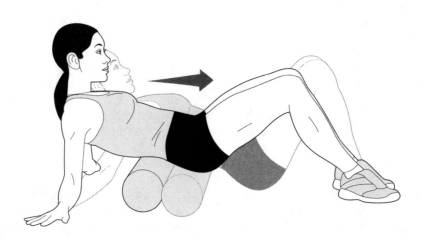

SIDE PLANK

• Lie on your side and use your forearm to support your body.

• Raise your hips until your body forms a straight line from shoulder to ankles. Hold for 30 seconds, then repeat for the other side.

BIRD DOG

• Get down on your hands and knees with your palms flat on the floor and shoulder-width apart.

• Brace your core and raise your right arm and left leg until they're in line with your body. Hold for 10 to 15 seconds.

• Return to the starting position. Repeat with your left arm and right leg. Continue to alternate for 10 reps.

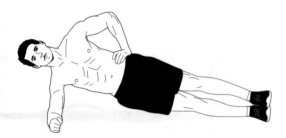

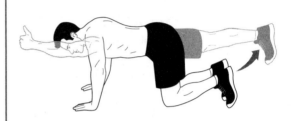

SWISS-BALL STIR-THE-POT

• Kneel in front of a Swiss ball and rest your forearms, parallel, on the ball, and make fists. Brace your core and hold.

• While keeping your back straight, move the ball in a tight circle with your forearms, as if you're stirring a pot. If your back begins to break form, your rotations are too big. Do 5 to 8 rotations, then reverse rotation direction and repeat.

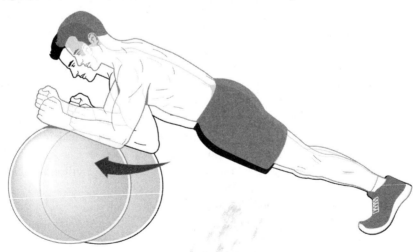

THE PROBLEM:
Hip Pain

THE SYMPTOMS: Pain can flare up virtually anywhere around your hip joint: in the groin area, on the bump on the outside of your hip, in the front of your hip, or around the gluteus muscles in the back. The pain can be dull or sharp and flare up at different times.

WHAT'S GOING ON: As with the shoulder joint, there are lots of moving parts that can throw things off kilter in the hip: the labrum (a cartilage cushion inside the joint); the articular cartilage on the surface of the bones; the iliopsoas muscle, which flexes the hip forward; the gluteus muscles, which extend it backward; and the tensor fascia lata on the outside of the joint. Then there are the bones themselves—the femur, the largest bone in your body, and acetabulum, the socket of the hip joint inside your ilium, or hip bone.

Pain in different areas of the hip joint can signal different injuries or conditions: A dull, achy pain that flares up at night or in the morning generally signals arthritis; pain in the groin can indicate a possible stress fracture, a torn labrum, or impingement of the iliopsoas; pain on the outside of the hip can signal a pinching or irritation of the bursa, a fluid-filled sac that cushions the

outside edge of the femur bone.

Several other conditions can lead to hip pain, including:

- **Tendinitis** in the iliotibial (IT) band on the outside of the thigh

- **Osteonecrosis,** a degenerative condition of the bones

- **Disc Herniation** and sciatica

- **Hip Fracture,** often as a result of osteoporosis, or loss of bone density

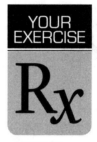

YOUR EXERCISE

Joints are stabilized by two major mechanisms: passive structures (bones and ligaments) and active ones (muscles). The stability provided by bones and ligaments is known as *static stability,* and the stability that muscles provide is called *dynamic stability.*

Loss of static stability can result from a number of causes: injury, overuse or underuse, and arthritis among them. The good news is that you can make up for a loss of static stability by improving the strength and coordination of the muscles surrounding your joints. Get stronger, in other words, and many of your symptoms will most likely improve—without drugs, surgery, or arduous rehab.

The most important muscles to strengthen around the hip joint are the glutes—your butt muscles, which work to extend your hip joint from the flexed position (knee toward your chest) to the fully extended position (leg kicked back behind you). Weakness in these muscles—the largest ones in your body—is common, even among some active people, because of all the sitting we do, and often leads to other issues, including hamstring tears and lower-back pain. I have a saying: "A strong butt is the key to a happy life!"

See "The Hip-Saving Workout" starting on the next page.

When to Call a Doctor

When your gait, or the mechanics of your walking, have changed noticeably (as in a limp), it's a good sign you should see a doctor: You're compensating for some pretty severe pain. Also pay attention to pain that gradually gets worse with time and doesn't respond to home-treatment methods like stretching, over-the-counter anti-inflammatory medication, ice, or "The Hip-Saving Workout," on the next page.

THE HIP-SAVING WORKOUT

Hip pain can originate from many sources—some serious, some less so. The best way to prevent hip trouble, or reduce minor hip pain? Get your butt moving—literally. The muscles of your buttocks play an enormous role in stabilizing and properly mobilizing your hip joint, as do the all-important core muscles. Fire them up and say good-bye to hip pain.

If any of the recommended exercises hurt, limit the range of motion: not so deep on the squats, not so hard on the stretches. Over time, the pain-free range should expand until you can perform all the moves comfortably over their full range.

FOAM ROLLING

If you've never foam-rolled before, be prepared. It's uncomfortable and can even be painful when you start. Don't worry—the more painful it is, the more that muscle needs foam rolling. The good news is that the more you do it, the less discomfort you'll feel. For each muscle that you work, slowly move the roller back and forth over it for 30 seconds. If you hit a really tender spot, pause on it for 5 to 10 seconds.

HAMSTRING ROLL

• Place a foam roller under your right knee, with your leg straight. Cross your left leg over your right ankle. Put your hands flat on the floor for support. Keep your back naturally arched.

• Roll your body forward until the roller reaches your glutes. Then roll back and forth. Repeat with the roller under your left thigh.

NOTE: If rolling one leg is too difficult, perform the movement with both legs on the roller.

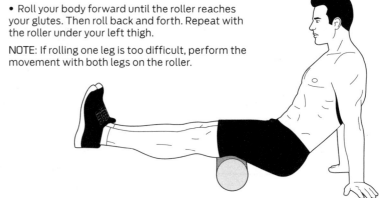

GLUTES ROLL

• Sit with a foam roller positioned on the back of your right thigh, just below your glutes. Cross your right leg over the front of your left thigh. Put your hands flat on the floor for support.

• Roll your body forward until the roller reaches your lower back. Then roll back and forth. Repeat with the roller under your left glute.

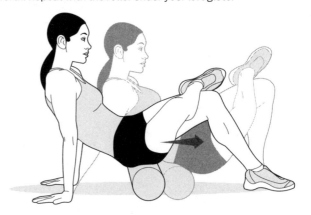

ILIOTIBIAL-BAND ROLL

• Lie on your right side and place your right hip on a foam roller. Put your right forearm on the floor for support. Cross your left leg over your right and place your left foot flat on the floor.

• Roll your body forward until the roller reaches your knee. Then roll back and forth. Lie on your left side and repeat with the roller under your left hip. (If this becomes too easy over time, place your left leg on top of your right instead of bracing it on the floor).

IMPORTANT NOTE:
Your iliotibial band—commonly called the IT band—is a tough strip of connective tissue that runs down the side of your thigh, starting on your hip bone and connecting just below your knee. When you start foam rolling, you'll probably find that this tissue is one of the most sensitive areas that you can roll over, perhaps due to the high tension of the band. Remember, pain means you need to roll it. Make this a priority, because over time, if your IT band is too tight, it could cause knee pain.

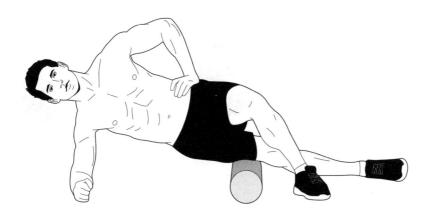

QUADRICEPS-AND-HIP-FLEXOR ROLL

• Lie facedown on the floor with a foam roller positioned above your right knee. Cross your left leg over your right ankle and place your elbows on the floor for support.

• Roll your body backward until the roller reaches the top of your right thigh. Then roll back and forth. Repeat with the roller under your left thigh. (If that's too hard, perform the movement with both thighs on the roller.)

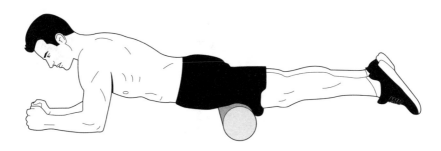

HIP-FRIENDLY EXERCISES

GLUTE BRIDGE (3 SETS OF 10)

Lie faceup on the floor with your knees bent and your feet flat on the floor. Place your arms out to your sides, your palms facing up. Raise your hips so your body forms a straight line from your shoulders to your knees. Squeeze your glutes as you raise your hips. Make sure you're pushing with your heels. To make it easier, you can position your feet so that your toes rise off the floor. Pause for 5 seconds in the up position, then lower your body back to the starting position.

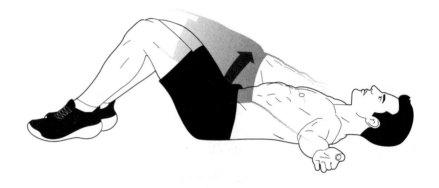

REAR-FOOT ELEVATED SPLIT SQUAT

1 SET OF 12 PER SIDE

Stand in a staggered stance, your left foot in front of your right 2 to 3 feet apart. Place just the instep of your back foot on a bench or chair. Pull your shoulders back and brace your core. Lower your body as deeply as you can, keeping your back foot on the bench. Keep your shoulders back and chest up through the movement. Pause, then return to the starting position. Halfway through the prescribed time, switch to the other foot.

BODY-WEIGHT SQUAT

1 SET OF 15 TO 20

Stand as tall as you can with your feet spread shoulder-width apart. Place your fingers on the back of your head (as if you have just been arrested). Pull your elbows and shoulders back and stick out your chest. Lower your body as far as you can by pushing your hips back and bending your knees. Pause, then slowly push yourself back to the starting position.

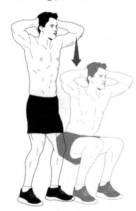

PLANK

Get into pushup position, but bend your elbows and rest your weight on your forearms. Your body should form a straight line from your shoulders to your ankles. Brace your core and hold for 30 seconds.

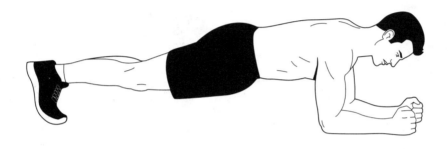

SIDE PLANK

Lie on your side and use your forearm to support your body. Raise your hips until your body forms a straight line from shoulder to ankles. Hold for 30 seconds and repeat for the other side.

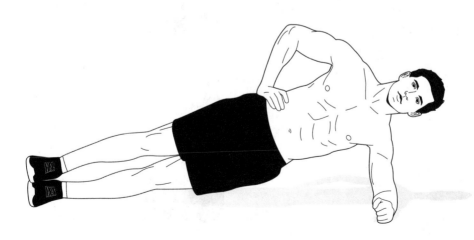

STRETCHES

Hold each for
30 seconds
per side.

BUTTERFLY STRETCH

Sit on the floor, bend your knees,
slide your feet toward your and
place the soles of your feet
together. Keeping your chest up
and your lower back in its
natural arch, drop your knees as
far as you can toward the floor.
If necessary, place your hands
on the floor behind you for
balance. Hold for 30 seconds.

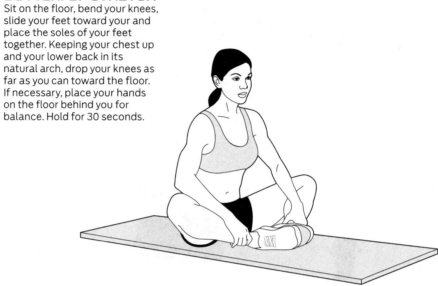

SEATED TWIST

Sit upright with the soles of
your feet together, knees
spread wide. Step your right
foot across the left and place
it flat on the floor near the
outside of your left knee.
Keeping your back straight,
your right foot on the floor,
and your right knee pointing
toward the ceiling, hug your
right knee with your left arm,
pull it toward your chest, and
rotate your upper body to the
right. Hold for 30 seconds
and repeat on the other side.

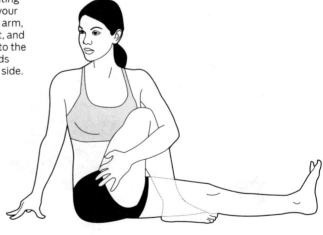

LYING DEAD BUG

Lie on your back and draw your knees up to your chest, allowing your knees to spread wider than your shoulders. Keeping your butt, shoulder blades, and the back of your head on the floor, reach between your feet, and grab the outer edge of the soles of your feet, palms facing inward, near your big toes (if you can't reach your feet, grab your ankles or calves). Hold for 30 seconds.

KNEELING QUAD/HIP FLEXOR STRETCH, LOWER LEG AGAINST THE WALL

• Assume a lunging position with your left foot forward, your right knee on the floor, and both knees at a 90-degree angle. Extend your right arm overhead. Keeping your torso upright, your hips and shoulders square, and your right knee on the floor, step your left foot forward about 12 inches and push your hips forward and downward until you feel a deep stretch in the front of your right hip. Hold for 30 seconds and repeat on the other side.

• Place a gym mat next to a wall. Face away from the wall and assume a kneeling lunge position on the pad with your left knee down and your right foot flat on the floor in front of you. Slide backward toward the wall, pointing the toes of your left foot toward the ceiling. Keeping your left knee on the floor, inch your foot up the wall behind you until you feel a comfortable stretch in the front of the left thigh. Place both hands on your right knee and extend your back into an upright posture. Hold for 30 seconds and repeat on the other side.

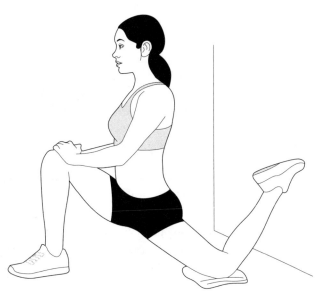

THE PROBLEM:
Knee Pain

THE SYMPTOMS: Well . . . your knee hurts. The pain can originate under or around the kneecap, or inside the joint itself. Additional symptoms include swelling, locking up or stiffening of the joint, or a sudden change in gait.

WHAT'S GOING ON: Your knee joint is like the middle child in a family of three: always taking the blame for everyone else's mistakes. When your knees hurt, it's often because of a problem in the joints above or below, rather than a problem in the knee itself: If your ankles and hips aren't adequately strong and flexible, your knee joints can suffer.

Contact sports and intense athletic training can cause ligament sprains in the knee, of course—I tore my ACL in medical school—but in many people, inactivity is an even more likely culprit: Long periods of sitting can accelerate wear and tear on the joint. And when a person doesn't exercise, the muscles around the knee joint weaken, causing instability and pain.

Knee pain can also be caused by problems in the alignment of the joint itself. Sometimes these issues are genetic (women are more prone to knee injury than men due to their wider hip structure); some-

times they are caused by a previous injury or long-term overuse.

Other causes of knee pain include more chronic conditions like tendinitis, bursitis, or arthritis. Being overweight or obese can exacerbate many of these problems by contributing to excessive strain on the joints.

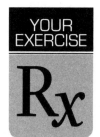

YOUR EXERCISE

I always recommend seeing a doctor for joint pain (see "When to Call a Doctor"). Follow your health care practitioner's guidelines for physical activity while recovering from a diagnosed joint condition or an acute injury to the knee.

If cleared for activity, your first priority should be to strengthen and stretch the muscles surrounding the hips, thighs, and ankles (see "The Knee-Saving Workout," page 130), and to get back into regular movement as quickly and safely as possible.

If obesity or inactivity contribute to your knee pain, it's essential that you find a way to exercise safely without reinjuring yourself or making your pain worse. At first, you can play around the pain, focusing most of your exercise on your upper body. As pain subsides, start incorporating low-impact activities: Swimming can be an excellent form of aerobic activity for people with joint pain; cycling, uphill walking, or using an elliptical trainer can also work well. Strength training, staying within a pain-free range of motion at all times, and using manageable weights at first, can also be a safe and effective way of regaining strength and function. Immediately stop any activity that sets off your knee pain.

When to Call a Doctor

As I mentioned, see a doctor for any kind of joint pain. But don't waste any time if you experience any of the following:

• You've experienced an acute injury to your knee, especially if you hear or feel a pop in the joint at the moment of impact.

• You experience any joint pain or swelling that lasts more than 48 hours.

• Your knee joint gives out frequently or appears to have lost range of motion.

THE KNEE-SAVING WORKOUT

The following workout will speed your recovery from a knee injury, help prevent further injury, and alleviate minor pain stemming from too much sitting *or* too much training. You can perform the workout as often as once a day, prior to other types of exercise:

FOAM ROLLING

If you've never foam-rolled before, be prepared. It's uncomfortable, and can even be painful when you start. Don't worry—the more painful it is, the more that muscle needs foam rolling. The good news is that the more you do it, the less discomfort you'll feel. For each muscle that you work, slowly move the roller back and forth over it for 30 seconds. If you hit a really tender spot, pause on it for 5 to 10 seconds.

CALF ROLL

• Place a foam roller under your right ankle, with your right leg straight. Cross your left leg over your right ankle. Put your hands flat on the floor for support and keep your back naturally arched.

• Roll your body forward until the roller reaches the back of your right knee. Then roll back and forth. Repeat with the roller under your left calf. (If this is too hard, perform the movement with both legs on the roller.)

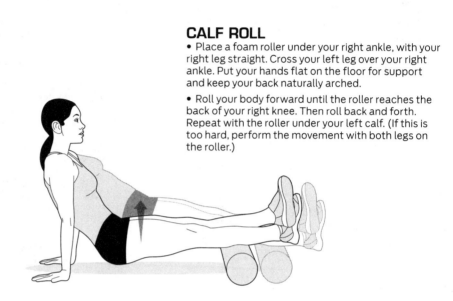

HAMSTRING ROLL

• Place a foam roller under your right knee, with your leg straight. Cross your left leg over your right ankle. Put your hands flat on the floor for support. Keep your back naturally arched.

• Roll your body forward until the roller reaches your glutes. Then roll back and forth. Repeat with the roller under your left thigh.

NOTE: If rolling one leg is too difficult, perform the movement with both legs on the roller.

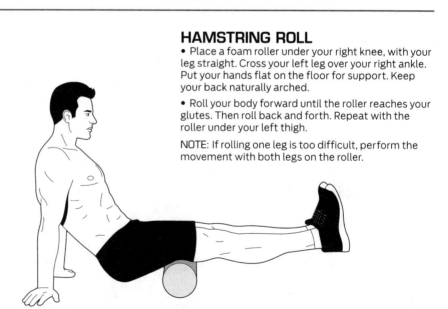

ILIOTIBIAL-BAND ROLL

• Lie on your right side and place your right hip on a foam roller. Put your right forearm on the floor for support. Cross your left leg over your right and place your left foot flat on the floor.

• Roll your body forward until the roller reaches your knee. Then roll back and forth. Lie on your left side and repeat with the roller under your left hip. (If this becomes too easy over time, place your left leg on top of your right instead of bracing it on the floor.)

IMPORTANT NOTE: Your iliotibial band—commonly called the IT band—is a tough strip of connective tissue that runs down the side of your thigh, starting on your hip bone and connecting just below your knee. When you start foam rolling, you'll probably find that this tissue is one of the most sensitive areas that you can roll over, perhaps due to the high tension of the band. Remember, pain means you need to roll it. Make this a priority, because over time, if your IT band is too tight, it could cause knee pain.

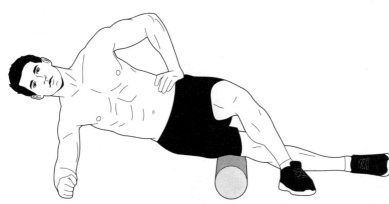

QUADRICEPS-AND-HIP-FLEXOR ROLL

• Lie facedown on the floor with a foam roller positioned above your right knee. Cross your left leg over your right ankle and place your elbows on the floor for support.

• Roll your body backward until the roller reaches the top of your right thigh. Then roll back and forth. Repeat with the roller under your left thigh. (If that's too hard, perform the movement with both thighs on the roller.)

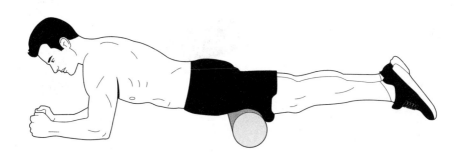

STRETCHES

Hold for
30-seconds
each.

KNEELING WALL STRETCH
(QUADRICEPS AND HIP FLEXOR)

Assume a lunging position with your left foot forward, your right knee on the floor, and both knees at a 90-degree angle. Extend your right arm overhead. Keeping your torso upright, your hips and shoulders square, and your right knee on the floor, step your left foot forward about 12 inches and push your hips forward and downward until you feel a deep stretch in the front of your right hip. Hold for 30 seconds and repeat on the other side.

Place a gym mat next to a wall. Face away from the wall and assume a kneeling lunge position on the pad with your left knee down and your right foot flat on the floor in front of you. Slide backward toward the wall, pointing the toes of your left foot toward the ceiling. Keeping your left knee on the floor, inch your foot up the wall behind you until you feel a comfortable stretch in the front of the left thigh. Place both hands on your right knee and extend your back into an upright posture. Hold for 30 seconds and repeat on the other side.

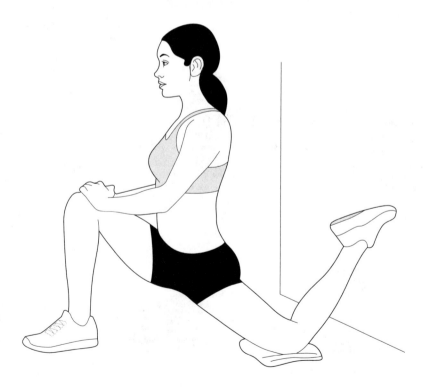

STRAIGHT-LEG CALF STRETCH

Stand about 2 feet in front of a wall in a staggered stance, left foot in front of your right. Place your hands on the wall and lean against it. Shift your weight to your back foot until you feel a stretch in your calf. Hold this stretch for 30 seconds on each side, then repeat twice for a total of 3 sets. Perform this routine daily, and up to 3 times a day if you're really tight.

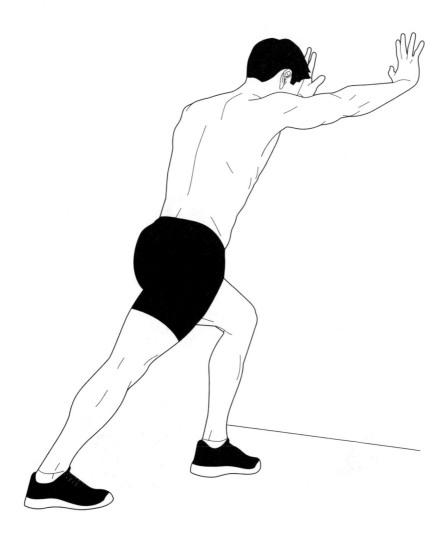

KNEE-FRIENDLY EXERCISES

SINGLE-LEG HIP BRIDGE
3 SETS OF 10 PER LEG

Lie faceup on the floor with your left knee bent and your right leg straight. Raise your right leg until it's in line with your left thigh. Place your arms out to your sides at 45-degree angles to your torso, palms facing up. Push your hips upward, keeping your right leg elevated and in line with your left thigh. Be sure to push up from your heel (you can raise your toes to help). Your body should form a straight line from your shoulders to your knees. Pause, then slowly lower your body and leg back to the starting position.

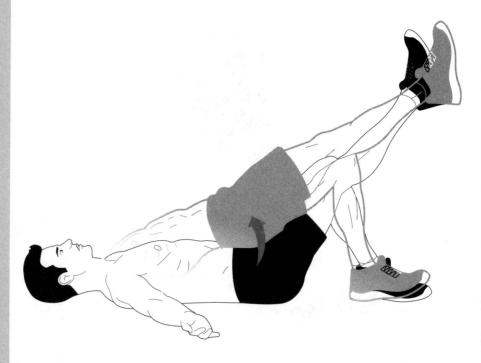

X-BAND WALK

3 TO 5 X 10 TO 15 PER LEG

Take hold of the handles on an elastic resistance band, allowing the center of the band to touch the floor. Stand on the center of the band, using a parallel, shoulder-width stance. Now exchange handles so that the handle in your right hand stretches toward the outside of your left foot and vice versa, and the band forms an "x" in front of you.

Hold the handles at waist level and pull the band taut. Keeping your chest high, your shoulders square, and your feet parallel, step laterally to your right 12 inches—first with your right foot, then with your left. Continue moving to your right for 15 steps, then repeat the exercise, moving to your left.

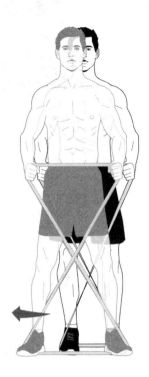

SINGLE-LEG STIFF-LEG DEADLIFT WALK

3 X 10 PER LEG

Stand with your feet hip-distance apart, arms at your sides. Shift your weight onto your right foot and lift your left foot a few inches off the floor. Keeping your back in its natural arch, your left leg and hip extended, and the toes of your left foot pointing toward the floor, begin to hinge forward on your right hip, simultaneously bending the right knee slightly. At the same time, extend your arms in front of you, elbows straight, palms facing one another. Continue hinging forward on your right hip until you are balancing on your right foot with your arms fully extended overhead, and your left leg, torso, and arms forming a straight line parallel to the floor (or as close as you can get without rounding your back or rolling to one side). Slowly return to an upright position, stepping forward with your left foot, and repeat on the other side. Alternate sides for the appropriate number of repetitions.

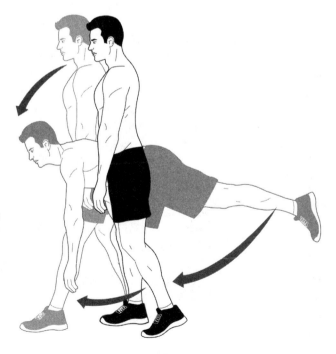

THE PROBLEM:
Neck and Shoulder Pain

THE SYMPTOMS: Your neck and shoulder . . . wait for it . . . hurt (4 years of med school, folks!). The feeling could be dull, achy, and continuous or sharp and sudden, caused when you assume a particular position with your arm or head.

WHAT'S GOING ON: Neck and shoulder pain are among the most common forms of orthopedic pain. In 2003, almost 14 million people saw a doctor for shoulder pain.

Why is this area so sensitive? For one thing, there are lots of moving parts, and therefore a lot that can go wrong: In order for your arm to cover a healthy range, lots of different structures get in on the act—not just the ball-and-socket (glenohumeral) joint of the shoulder itself, but your scapulae (shoulder blades), your clavicles (collarbones), your cervical vertebrae (spinal neck bones), and all the soft tissues around them that move those bones. Unlike your hip joints, the socket for the shoulder joint is fairly shallow, which allows you to reach and stretch in many directions, but also makes the joint more vulnerable to injury.

Common problems that sometimes bring on shoulder pain include arthritis, frozen shoulder (some-times caused by diabetes), tendinitis in the rotator cuff, impingement (compression or abrasion of the rotator cuff by bones or ligaments), pinched nerves, and injuries of all kinds, including fractures, dislocations and subluxations, sprain, and partial or complete tearing of the rotator cuff.

These days, though, probably the most common cause of shoulder and neck pain is good ol'-fashioned sitting. Long periods at a desk or on a couch can cause your head to drift forward, your upper back to round, and your shoulder blades to wing out from your spine. Stay in this position long enough and it becomes habitual—throwing your arms, neck, and shoulders out of their optimal alignment more or less permanently. Over time, this new position itself may cause pain. Or it may make you more susceptible to injury during exercise or sports activity. The misaligned vertebrae in your neck may also lead to a compressed nerve, leading to what can feel like shoulder or arm pain—even though the problem is in your neck.

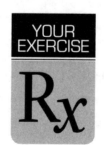

YOUR EXERCISE The best type of exercise for preventing and treating shoulder and neck pain is strength training. A 2008 Dutch study of female office workers with shoulder pain found that a regimen of five strength-training exercises—the one-arm row, shoulder abduction, shoulder elevation, reverse fly, and upright row— alleviated their pain symptoms by 50 percent. A comparable group of women doing a cycling program saw no such improvements.

For a complete shoulder-injury prevention-and-rehab workout— including useful stretches and foam-rolling techniques—see the next page.

When to Call a Doctor

If you've suffered an acute trauma to your shoulder, get yourself to a doctor. Depending on what's going on, you might need anything from immobilization to physical therapy to a steroid injection. If you're a desk-sitter and your pain is mild, however, try the exercises on the next page before making an appointment— you may be able to clear up your pain on your own.

NECK-FRIENDLY EXERCISES

Perform 3 sets of 12 reps for each exercise, except where noted.

SEATED DUMBBELL EXTERNAL ROTATION

Grab a dumbbell in your right hand and sit on a bench. Place your right foot on the bench with your knee bent. Bend your right elbow 90 degrees and place the inside portion of it on your right knee. Use your free hand for support. Without changing the bend in your elbow, and while keeping your wrist straight, rotate your upper arm and forearm up and back as far as you can. Pause, then return to the starting position. Perform the prescribed number of repetitions with your right arm, then switch and perform the same number with your left arm.

INVERTED ROW

Grab the bar above you with an overhand, shoulder-width grip. Hang with your arms completely straight and your hands positioned directly above your shoulders. Your body should form a straight line from your ankles to your head. Initiate the movement by pulling your shoulder blades back, then continue the pull with your arms to lift your chest to the bar. Pause, then slowly lower your body back to the starting position.

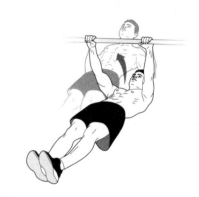

FLOOR Y-T-I RAISES
NOTE: Do 8 to 10 reps of each.

Y RAISE

Lie facedown on the floor. Allow your arms to rest on the floor, completely straight and at a 30-degree angle to your body, your palms facing each other (thumbs up). Your body should resemble the letter Y. Raise your arms as high as you can, pause, then slowly lower back to the starting position.

T RAISE

Lie facedown on the floor. Move your arms so they're out to your sides—perpendicular to your body with the thumb sides of your hands pointing up—and raise them as high as you can. Pause, then slowly lower back to the starting position.

I RAISE

Lie facedown on the floor. Position your arms straight above your shoulders so your body forms a straight line from your feet to your fingertips. Your palms should be facing each other, thumbs pointing up. Raise your arms as high as you can, pause, then slowly lower back to the starting position.

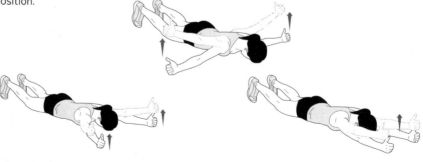

PULLUP

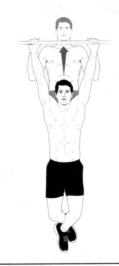

- If you can't get 12 reps, do as many as possible for 3 sets or assist yourself using a chair.

- Grab the pullup bar with a shoulder-width, overhand grip. Hang at arm's length. You should return to this position—known as a dead hang—each time you lower your body back down. Cross your ankles behind you. Pull your chest to the bar as you squeeze your shoulder blades together. Once the top of your chest touches the bar, pause, then slowly lower your body back to a dead hang.

SERRATUS CHAIR SHRUG

5-SECOND HOLDS

Sit upright on a chair or bench and place your hands flat on the sitting surface next to your hips. Completely straighten your arms. Allow your shoulders and back muscles to relax so your torso lowers between your shoulders. Your hips should just be off the edge of the bench. Press your shoulders down as you lift your upper body. Your torso should rise between your shoulders. Pause for 5 seconds, then lower your body back to the starting position.

NOTE: You can do this exercise at your desk or even on your couch while you watch TV.

INVERTED SHOULDER PRESS

(3 SETS, AS MANY REPS AS POSSIBLE)

- Assume a pushup position, but place your feet on a bench or chair and push your hips up so that your torso is nearly perpendicular to the floor. Your hands should be slightly wider than your shoulders and your arms should be straight.

- Without changing your body posture, lower your body until your head nearly touches the floor. Pause, then return to the starting position by pushing your body back up until your arms are straight.

NOTE: While the inverted shoulder press is technically a pushup, the tweak to your form shifts more of the workload to your shoulders and triceps, reducing the demand on your chest.

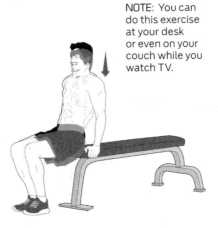

WHAT *NOT* TO DO WHEN YOUR SHOULDERS HURT

Sometimes injury prevention and pain relief are as much about what *not* to do as what to do. As always, avoid *any* exercise that causes immediate, noticeable pain—that's a no-brainer. Outside of that, though, here are some exercises that might be causing or exacerbating your shoulder pain, and what you should be doing instead:

- **Don't do:** Behind-the-neck press
Substitute: Dumbbell overhead press

- **Don't do:** Behind-the-neck pulldown or pullup
Substitute: Pulldowns or pullups to the front, neutral grip (hands facing each other)

- **Don't do:** Upright row
Substitute: Barbell or dumbbell shrugs

- **Don't do:** Barbell back squats
Substitute: Barbell or kettlebell front squat, overhead squat, plyometric (explosive) squat

THE PROBLEM:
Osteoarthritis

THE SYMPTOM: Your weight-bearing joints—namely your hips, knees, and spine—are inflamed and painful, and the joints in your thumb, neck, and big toe may be as well. The pain and stiffness usually get worse with excessive or repetitive movement, overuse, or long periods of inactivity or rest. The middle and end joints of your fingers may be enlarged and swollen, though these areas may or may not be painful.

WHAT'S GOING ON: Osteoarthritis, or OA, affects cartilage—the firm, rubbery, shock-absorbing material that covers the ends of your bones. When you have OA, the cartilage in your knees and hips becomes stiff and loses its spring and can wear away in some areas, like a bald patch on a tire. Ligaments and tendons stretch and deform to compensate, causing you pain. If the condition worsens, the bones can rub against one another.

Some 27 million Americans have OA. Most adults over 60 have some degree of OA, though it also can set in as early as your twenties. Women are five times as likely to have OA as men.

Risk factors for OA include age, heredity, previous overuse injury to the affected area, a preexisting case of rheumatoid arthritis, and obesity—which significantly increases wear and tear on weight-bearing joints.

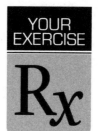

I say it often: Strength controls pain. Exercise improves osteoarthritis symptoms by helping you lose weight so that the pressure on your joints is reduced, and by strengthening the muscles around the joints—so your bone surfaces absorb less of pressure.

If you have OA, exercise may feel like the last thing you want to do—but do it! Research indicates that inactivity may actually cause cartilage to atrophy (thin out)—a situation that you'll definitely want to avoid.

For OA, I recommend a continuum of exercise based on your symptoms and severity of pain. Once your symptoms improve, step up to the next level:

• **FOR INTENSE PAIN** (difficulty with many everyday tasks most of the time): swimming and/or water aerobics, strength training, and stretching (see "The Arthritis Strength-Building Plan" on page 142)

- **FOR MILD PAIN** (some pain after sitting, resting, or lots of activity): swimming, walking, brisk walking if tolerated, basic strength training with more intensity

- **FOR OCCASIONAL, MILD PAIN** (infrequent, mild pain): Cleared for all activity except jogging, running, and other high-impact sports. Keep weight down and strength up to avoid symptoms returning or worsening.

When to Call a Doctor

If you have osteoarthritis symptoms, your doctor should know about it. You can probably manage mild symptoms at home with exercise and judicious use of NSAIDs (nonsteroidal anti-inflammatory drugs like Advil and Motrin). If symptoms don't respond or get worse, your health care provider may do an x-ray and/or MRI of the affected joints and proceed from there, perhaps prescribing a stronger anti-inflammatory or a steroid injection into the joint itself.

Physical and occupational therapy can provide relief from day-to-day symptoms and give you strategies on how to avoid making your OA worse.

Unfortunately, no medical treatment currently available can reverse OA symptoms or directly slow degeneration caused by OA. But that doesn't mean you're out of luck: The best medicine for OA is the best medicine, period—weight loss and smart exercise.

THE ARTHRITIS STRENGTH-BUILDING PLAN

You've got osteoarthritis, and you know you should exercise. But everything hurts. What's a person with creaky knees to do? Don't fret, and don't stay on the couch: You'll only make things worse.

Water-based workouts can be great—for the first few weeks. But your first line of defense should be resistance exercise. Why? With strength training, you can control the amount of pressure you put on a joint—and gradually increase it as your symptoms get better. That's not true of most other types of exercise—even walking. Try these moves two or three times a week for a month. If your knees or hips start to hurt during exercise, back off and do less. Hold each stretch for 30 seconds; on strength-training moves (see page 144), do 2 to 4 sets of 10 reps, moving slowly throughout the exercise.

STRETCHES

OVERHEAD LAT STRETCH
• Stand upright in a shoulder-width stance, feet parallel.

• Interlace your fingers, turn your palms away from you, straighten your arms, and extend them overhead. Breathe deeply and hold for 30 seconds.

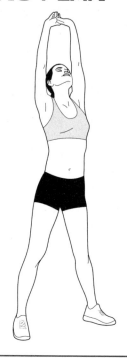

STRAIGHT-LEG CALF STRETCH
• Stand about 2 feet in front of a wall in a staggered stance, your left foot in front of your right. Place your hands on the wall and lean against it.

• Shift your weight to your back foot until you feel a stretch in your calf. Hold this stretch for 30 seconds on each side, then repeat twice for a total of 3 sets.

• Perform this routine daily, and up to 3 times a day if you're really tight.

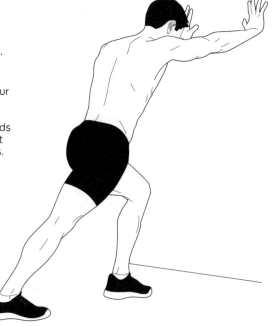

QUAD STRETCH

• From a standing position, bend your left knee so you can grab your left ankle with your left hand.

• Keeping your hips and shoulders square and your left knee pointing toward the floor, pull your left heel toward your butt until you feel a stretch in the front of your right thigh. Hold for 30 seconds and repeat on the other side.

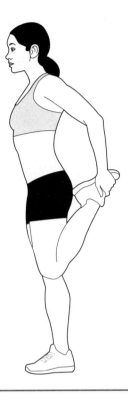

FORWARD BEND (YOGA)

Stand with your feet together, arms at your sides. Exhale as you bend forward at your hips, reaching your hands toward the floor. Imagine folding your body in half.

NOTE: For beginners, bend as far as you can and hold for 30 seconds, making sure to breathe slowly and deeply.

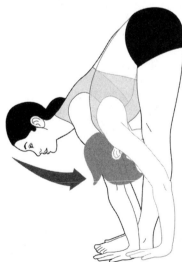

STRENGTH TRAINING

PRISONER SQUAT

Stand as tall as you can with your feet spread shoulder-width apart. Place your fingers on the back of your head (as if you have just been arrested). Pull your elbows and shoulders back, and stick out your chest. Lower your body as far as you can by pushing your hips back and bending your knees. Pause, then slowly push yourself back to the starting position.

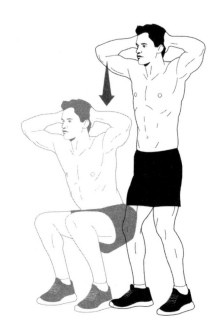

OVERHEAD DUMBBELL SQUAT

Stand with your feet slightly wider than hip-width apart. Hold a pair of dumbbells straight over your shoulders, your arms completely straight. Brace your core and lower your body as far as you can by pushing your hips back and bending your knees. Pause, then slowly push yourself back to the starting position.

NOTE: Keep your torso as upright as possible and don't let the dumbbells fall forward as you squat.

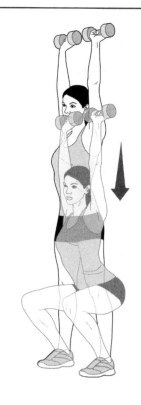

DUMBBELL LUNGE

• Grab a pair of dumbbells and hold them at arm's length next to your sides, your palms facing each other.

• Brace your core, step forward with your left leg, and slowly lower your body until your front knee is bent at least 90 degrees. Pause, then push yourself to the starting position as quickly as you can.

• Complete the prescribed number of repetitions with your left leg, then do the same number with your right leg.

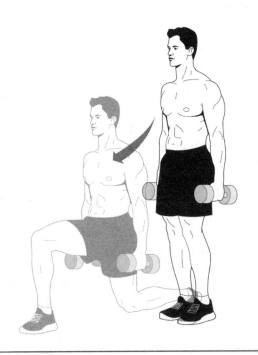

LOW SIDE-TO-SIDE LUNGE
(DUMBBELLS OPTIONAL)

• Stand with your feet set about twice shoulder-length apart, your feet facing straight ahead.

• Shift your weight over to your right leg as you push your hips backward and lower your body by dropping your hips and bending your knees. Your lower right leg should remain nearly perpendicular to the floor. Your left foot should remain flat on the floor.

• Without raising yourself back up to a standing position, reverse the movement to the left. Alternate back and forth.

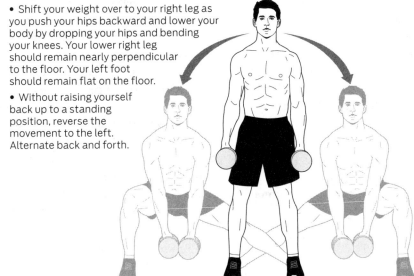

LEAN BODY, HAPPY JOINTS

Many people are overweight. Folks also tend to put on weight as they age. But if you're at risk for arthritis, such as from a previous knee injury, or if you have arthritis already, drop whatever weight you don't need, especially as you get older. The math is simple: The less weight you have to carry around, the less your joints have to bear. A lean physique also makes whatever strength gains you make that much more effective at supporting your joints.

One of my biggest goals as a doctor is helping you do everything you can to avoid a cancer diagnosis.

"Cancer" is a terrifying term. It covers a large array of illnesses, ranging from virulent brain tumors to slow-growing cancers you can live with for decades. That's part of why the disease is so tough to fight: It's mutable and comes in many forms.

And I'll be the first to admit that cancer absolutely cannot be cured with exercise. Even the most disciplined athletes in the world still get cancer.

But, the data on certain types of cancer show that exercise can be preventive. Recent studies suggest that regular exercise reduces many of the general markers of inflammation that are suspected in the development of certain types of cancer.

In this special section, I'm going to present the case for why exercise *is* extremely important, and effective, in preventing certain cancers—even if it doesn't offer guarantees. I'll also address how the right approach to exercise can help enormously in the *treatment* and *recovery* from cancer.

EXERCISE AND CANCER PREVENTION

Since cancer starts at a localized point—a skin lesion or a tumor, for example—it can appear to be a localized problem. That's true to a certain degree (and why you can surgically remove some cancers), but more and more health care professionals are treating cancer as a systemic disease, that is, symptomatic of a whole-body failure. It makes sense, then, to try to bolster all components of a person's health—emotional, psychological, and spiritual as well as physical—in approaching cancer prevention and treatment.

Research is showing that exercise, which addresses many if not all of these dimensions, is one very effective way of doing this.

The Copenhagen Male Study, a longitudinal research project that tracked health outcomes for 5,000 Danish men for 23 years, found that men who exercised—even moderately—were significantly less likely than nonexercisers to develop intestinal cancer. Other large-scale studies have shown similar outcomes with cancer of the esophagus and colon in both sexes, and with breast and endometrial cancers in women. And exercise very likely plays a role in the prevention of many other cancers as well, including prostate, testicular, ovarian, uterine, lung, and non-Hodgkin's lymphoma.

One massive study, published in 2012 and following more than 65,000 volunteers, showed that regular physical activity decreased people's risk of hematologic cancers (blood, lymph nodes, bone marrow).

How does this work? It may be related to other factors—people who exercise are more likely to eat a good diet, get better sleep, have higher fitness and lower body weight, and take other self-care measures. In the digestive tract, it's most likely because exercise keeps food and waste material moving through the system so that cancer doesn't have a chance to take hold. And the balancing effects of exercise on your endocrine system, including both male and female sex hormones, probably helps prevent cancers of the testes, prostate, and breast.

Overall, though, it's probably because exercise simply ups your game, internally and externally. Your immune system works better. Cardiovascular and pulmonary function improve. Your energy goes up. There's barely a cell in your body that doesn't kick up its performance a notch in response to regular exercise. It's a head-to-toe engine flush, and so far, that's about as good an explanation as anyone has about how exercise helps prevent cancer.

EXERCISE AND CANCER TREATMENT

If you or someone you know gets hit with a diagnosis, the crucial first step is finding and working with a good team of doctors on medical treatment for the disease. Outside of that, though, there are a host of complementary treatments that have been shown to be effective not only in combating the disease itself but in fighting off some of the worst side effects of cancer and cancer treatment, including depression, weakness, and fatigue. Some of these treatments include acupuncture, massage, meditation, and group counseling. And, increasingly, oncologists are encouraging patients to use mild to moderate exercise such as walking, swimming, and light weight training to help alleviate the side effects of cancer treatment. One other possibility: Exercise's anti-inflammatory properties. Chronic inflammation in the body is associated with many chronic diseases. A 2013 study showed that regular physical activity reduces low-grade inflammation in the body.

A 2008 research review found that, across the board, exercise may increase survival rates following a cancer diagnosis by up to 60 percent. A second study found that, in women recovering from breast cancer treatment, a combined program of aerobic and resistance training produced "large and rapid improvements in health-related outcomes." A third study, this one from 2012, found that people with advanced-stage cancer who exercised had lower levels of psychological anxiety, stress, and depression, and improved levels of physical pain, fatigue, shortness of breath, constipation, and insomnia.

Among these other benefits, working out also helps people with cancer minimize the risk of contracting other illnesses while undergoing cancer treatment. Some hormone therapies for breast and prostate cancer, for example, can substantially increase a person's risk of contracting cardiovascular disease, obesity, and type 2 diabetes—making treatment almost as much of a threat to a patient's health as the cancer itself. Appropriate exercise may be one of the best ways to help manage and treat these secondary diseases.

In the end, though, exercise may work best as an insurance policy that not only helps you prevent chronic disease like cancer, but gives you a stronger foundation of health from which to fight disease should you happen to contract it. Alwyn Cosgrove, whom I've mentioned before, is a former world champion martial artist, fitness author, and a very successful gym owner. He's also a two-time stage-IV cancer survivor.

As part of his treatment, Cosgrove had a stem cell transplant, which involves, essentially, wiping out a patient's immune system with chemotherapy, then replacing it with healthy stem cells.

Before getting cleared for the procedure, however, a stem-cell transplant candidate has to pass a series of fitness tests to make sure his body is up for it. Former champion athlete and diligent exerciser that he was, Cosgrove passed the tests with flying colors. He got through the procedure and beat the disease into remission—where it's stayed now for more than 6 years.

A huge success story, to be sure.

While in recovery, however, Cosgrove met a number of people who were trying to raise their fitness levels *in preparation* for the same procedure. He admired their dedication, but wondered how they'd be able to pull it off while fighting through both cancer and its strength-sapping treatments. How could a person *improve* their fitness under such circumstances? "Getting in shape is an uphill battle for everyone," he later said, "but cancer patients are starting well behind the starting blocks."

It's possible. People have done it. But it's tough.

Of course, you don't want to spend your life worrying about, or preparing for, life-threatening illness. But yet one more reason to have an exercise habit in place is as an insurance policy if, God forbid, you ever *do* come down with such an illness. Time and time again, we see that people who are in good physical shape going in make faster and more complete recovery from disease than those who aren't.

Maybe it's because people who are fit have more resilient immune systems. Maybe they're used to bouncing back from suffering, and have internal fortitude to spare. As with prevention and treatment, it's not entirely clear *why* being in shape helps a person get back on their feet after a major health crisis—just that it does.

"I knew that I had survived in part because when the disease hit me, I was in condition," concludes Cosgrove. "I was strong. I had muscle. I had cardio fitness. I had grit my teeth through tough strength training and running workouts. My body could handle whatever the doctors were going to throw at me. Cancer couldn't."

GENERAL GUIDELINES:

• **Avoid exercise** if you are experiencing extreme fatigue, anemia, or ataxia (loss of motor control).

• **Allow adequate time** to heal following surgery—as long as 8 weeks, depending on instructions from your health care provider.

• **During treatment,** chemotherapy and radiation can compromise the immune system, so take extra care that your workout environment is as clean as possible (home gym as opposed to public gym).

• **Some therapies** can leave patients with an increased risk of heart attack following treatment. Ask your doctors about this and modify cardiovascular exercise parameters accordingly.

• **Patients with bone metastases** (tumors) may need to modify exercise duration, intensity, and frequency to lower chances of fractures.

PREVENTION

Most studies of exercise for cancer prevention indicate that moderate exercise is probably all you need to lower your risk of many cancers. However, that may be because large, long-term studies often don't include many subjects who exercise more vigorously on a regular basis. Those that do actually suggest that people who are more continuously active—farmers, postal workers, and others who walk a lot as part of their job, for example—have an even lower risk of contracting cancer. If moderate exercise is all that you can handle, you'll certainly get at least some protection—but if you can do even more, so much the better.

TREATMENT AND RECOVERY

In 2010, the American College of Sports Medicine assembled a roundtable of thirteen experts to conduct an extensive review of the clinical studies to date on exercise for cancer survivors. Their conclusion:

Historically, clinicians advised cancer patients to rest and to avoid activity; however, emerging research on exercise has challenged this recommendation. The roundtable concluded that exercise training is safe during and after cancer treatments and results in improvements in physical functioning, quality of life, and cancer-related fatigue in several cancer survivor groups. Implications for disease outcomes and survival are still unknown.

SPECIAL SECTION
Cancer—*Continued*

Nevertheless, the benefits to physical functioning and quality of life are sufficient for the recommendation that cancer survivors follow the 2008 Physical Activity Guidelines for Americans, with specific exercise programming adaptations based on disease and treatment-related adverse effects. The advice to "avoid inactivity," even in cancer patients with existing disease or undergoing difficult treatments, is likely helpful.

In other words: Go for it. At the end of the day, you'll minimize side effects, heal faster, and feel better by exercising (with adaptations to suit your specific condition) than by resting completely.

Depending on what phase and type of treatment you're in, it may be possible to continue with, or even initiate, a rigorous exercise program. In some cases, even very mild exercise may seem like a Herculean task. You'll definitely want to work with your doctor on how much and what type of exercise is appropriate. But if you're cleared for exercise and struggling to get off the couch, know that working out itself may be effective in fighting off CRF (cancer-related fatigue), one of the more debilitating side effects of the disease. So the toughest step you take will probably be your first one.

EXERCISE AND SPECIFIC CANCERS

The ACSM offers the following guidelines for people recovering from different types of cancer:

BREAST CANCER:

• Women who have had surgery affecting the chest, arms, or shoulders should train around these areas until any limitations are resolved: Train the legs, core, and cardiovascular system. Train arms and shoulders in a manner that feels comfortable and feels safe. Should swelling, pain, or any changes in symptoms occur, see a doctor.

• Women with lymphedema (swelling caused by obstruction in the lymph nodes) should wear a well-fitting compression garment during exercise.

• Women undergoing hormone therapy or who have been diagnosed with osteoporosis or bony metastases may need to limit high-impact, weight-bearing activities and sports due to increased risk of fracture.

COLON CANCER:

• Patients with ostomy should seek permission from a physician before participating in contact sports or strength training, due to risk of blow to surgery site, possible infection, and hernia.

GYNECOLOGIC CANCER:

• Women with swelling or inflammation in the lower body or abdomen should seek medical care and train around these areas until these limitations are resolved. Work the upper body, ideally with a combination of strength training (weight machines are probably safest, to avoid straining in the abdominal wall) and cardiovascular exercise (using upper-body aerobic devices, such as the upper-body recumbent bike). Train the lower body to the extent that it feels comfortable and feels safe.

• Women with lymphedema (swelling caused by obstruction in the lymph nodes) should wear a well-fitting compression garment during exercise.

• Women undergoing hormone therapy, or who have been diagnosed with osteoporosis or bony metastases may need to limit high-impact, weight-bearing activities and sports due to increased risk of fracture.

HEMATOLOGIC CANCER (BLOOD, LYMPH NODES, BONE MARROW)—NO HSCT (STEM-CELL TRANSPLANT):

• Patients with multiple myeloma who have not received a stem-cell transplant have an increase risk of bone fracture, and may need to limit high-impact, weight-bearing activities and sports due to increased risk of fracture.

PROSTATE CANCER:

• Men who have had prostate cancer treatments may have an elevated risk of fractures and should consult their doctor about the need to limit high-impact, weight-bearing activities and sports.

• Patients with ostomy should also avoid excessive intra-abdominal pressure (common during lifting, straining, or breath holding).

PART 3

The Go-for-the-Gold Workout Program

U p to now I've talked about how exercise can help prevent and heal disease. As you've been reading, you may have been thinking, *Well, this is great, but I'm not sure where to start.* Or maybe you know where to start, or have already started, but are looking for new and challenging ideas. No matter what you're looking for, this section will help you. It's loaded with ideas for every type of exercise out there.

Or . . . maybe you want a complete, from-day-one body (and life-) changing fitness program. Well, this section gives you that, too. I can take you from completely sedentary to totally fit over a tailor-made time period. Four weeks? Yes. Three months? Of course. In fact, if you worked the entire section from beginning to end, you'd have constantly changing and fun workouts for *9 months*.

Yes, I'm serious about my exercise! But here's the best part about this section: You can adapt this information to any variation that works for you. The secret to exercise, after all, is exercising, and the best workout is one you never miss.

Get ready to have some fun. . . .

How to Get the Most Out of Every Workout

Before we jump into the first workouts, I want to offer some important guidelines on how to approach this program—and any exercise program you embark on from this day forward. The fact is, there are a million and one ways out there to improve your fitness, and a few thousand more, it seems, being born every day. Your choices are pretty close to infinite. But if you apply the following principles—I call them the "Ten Commandments of Fitness"—to any fitness endeavor you do, you can't go wrong.

THE TEN COMMANDMENTS OF FITNESS

1. Thou Shalt Have Fun. If you despise resistance training, or hate to run, all my preaching about the virtues of body-weight training or the joys of a Sunday morning 20-miler won't change your mind. So the first rule is to find something you enjoy.

Now, if you have specific fitness goals—say, losing lots of weight fast, gaining muscle, or getting stronger in a hurry, you're going to want to do a program tailored to help you reach those goals. We'll get into those specifics in this section. But if you don't enjoy—or learn to enjoy—those types of workouts, you probably won't stick with them, and you should find something else to do. An exercise program is only as good as the effort you put into it—and the joy you get out of it.

Maybe you've always wanted to explore dance or the martial arts or sculling or fencing or Ultimate Frisbee. Maybe golf or tennis sounds appealing. Or you could start über-simple and begin a walking program with a few friends. It's up to you.

Bottom line: Jump in and have fun.

2. Thou Shalt Set Goals.

You've heard this one before: The clearer and more explicit your goals, the more likely you are to accomplish them. That's as true about fitness as it is for your career and life in general.

So what are yours? The SMART acronym for strategic goal-setting, originally coined by George Doran in the 1980s, is a good way to start. To maximize your chances of success, your chosen goal should be *Specific, Measurable, Attainable, Relevant,* and *Time-Bound.* So make it something concrete: "Run a 5-K by July" is better than "feel better." Your goal should be challenging, but not unattainable: If you're a beginner, don't choose "walk 5 minutes this month," but don't choose "win Olympic gold in 2016," either. You should know when you've attained it, care about it, and give yourself a realistic time frame in which to pull it off.

For some people reading this book, walking for a half hour a day in three 10-minute segments, three times a week for the next month would be a terrific goal. Other readers may need something loftier, like bench-pressing 250 by your birthday. Every year on January first, trainer Alwyn Cosgrove—a gym owner, cancer survivor, and martial arts champion—resolves to do 250 workouts during the year. Given his schedule, age, and physical condition, that's a perfect goal. For you, it might be too much or too little. The goal is always specific to *you*.

And yes, what you've heard is true: Writing your goal down somewhere really does help.

3. Thou Shalt Work Hard.

Don't worry about this one if you're just getting started. For the first few weeks, all that matters is that you make exercising an enjoyable habit. But after that initial break-in period, if you're not pushing yourself at least a little bit a few times a week—by walking a little farther or faster, lifting a little more weight, or doing a few more pushups than you're used to—you're missing out on some of the most important benefits of exercise. One 2006 study, for example, found that people who exercised vigorously were significantly less likely to suffer heart attacks than moderate exercisers.

If you're new to exercise, *working hard* at something that's supposed to be *fun* may sound contradictory. You'll have to take me a bit on faith here, but hard workouts *are* fun. It might not be a type of fun you're used to, but once you're into the rhythm of it, you'll find that hard exercise is satisfying and invigorating, and you'll look forward to the jump in mental and physical energy it gives you. I see this in my students all the time: They walk into my weekend fitness classes feeling apprehensive, and they walk out glowing.

Personally, when I work out, I'm having the time of my life—even on mile 20 of the marathon stage of the Ironman, when every muscle fiber in my body is screaming at me to stop. It doesn't get any better than that!

4. Thou Shalt Not Be Bored.

One reason I enjoy training for multisport races is that it's always changing. Tired of swimming? Not to worry, you'll be on the bike soon. Saddle sore? There's a run coming up.

But you don't have to take your program to the extremes that I do to keep it interesting for yourself. If you get bored doing an activity you typically enjoy, take it as a sign that you may be burning out or courting injury. At the very least, you've stopped improving and are simply spinning your wheels.

Some experts recommend working out seasonally to stave off boredom and overwork: cross-country skiing in the winter and swimming in the summer, for example. Others prefer to switch activities when the mood strikes them: Fitness levels stay high, overworked areas of your body get a break, and underworked areas get a new training stimulus.

The result is new muscle, new skills, and new enthusiasm.

5. Thou Shalt Go Outside.

When we were kids, we understood this intuitively: We'd head out the door and start running, jumping, and climbing. Since then, we've been conditioned to exercise indoors, on bulky, expensive machines that dictate our movements for us. No wonder people learn to dread exercise.

Gyms do have advantages: They're convenient, especially when it's cold, wet, and dark outside; some offer great classes with inspiring, knowledgeable instructors; and the right equipment at the right time can definitely bring some novelty to a tired workout. But mounting evidence suggests that going outside at least some of the time adds something important to your workout. For one thing, it's a change from the indoors, where most of us spend lots of time already. For another, there are measurable fitness advantages to being outside: A soft, uneven trail run conditions your ankles and feet in ways that a flat, unchanging treadmill doesn't, and a real bike ride up real hills works your legs and cardio system better than even the most amped-up spinning instructor ever could.

Then there are more intangible benefits: A 2011 study found that "compared with exercising indoors, exercising in natural environments was associated with greater feelings of revitalization, increased energy

THE EXERCISE SECRET PRO ATHLETES KNOW

If you can understand this one little-known fact about exercise and your body, you'll be well on your way to making sure you maximize each workout and build a physique that performs better and resists injury. And it's all about two words: kinetic chain.

Your kinetic chain is basically your entire body from the top of your neck down to your toenails, one big interconnected chain of muscles, ligaments, tendons, bones, and so on. If you neglect to train one link of that chain, you then have a weak link. The result? You guessed it: a body part that underperforms and is vulnerable to injury.

For a majority of the sports injury cases I see in my office, whether the patient is 8 or 80, an improperly trained kinetic chain is to blame. As I tell my patients, "A healthy kinetic chain depends on both strength and flexibility. If you train your entire body, the whole chain, everything will feel better."

This is why I encourage total-body training and a variety of workouts that challenge new areas of your kinetic chain. Distance running is terrific exercise, but if that's all you do, eventually some links in your chain will break (usually when you're asking your runner's body to do something it's not conditioned to do).

Train the whole chain. Your body will reward you for it.

and positive engagement, together with decreases in tension, confusion, anger and depression."

So if you want an added mental and physical boost—and the weather is cooperating—take it outside.

6. Thou Shalt Listen to Thy Body.

This is probably one of the toughest ones to get right, especially when you're new to exercise. Your body is constantly giving you feedback about its need for food, water, rest, and movement. Sometimes those signals come through loud and clear; other times they're subtle. You need to start paying attention to the cues your body is sending you about when to push and when to back off.

When you first begin an exercise program, though, everything feels unusual, so you might suspect a serious injury when all you're feeling is normal muscle soreness. Soon enough, though, you'll be able tell the slightly achy feeling you get when a workout is working (and you can continue) from the sharp, intense pain of a real tweak (and you shouldn't).

On the other hand, you'll also come to know those days when you're up for an especially challenging workout—when you can take the long way home on your bike ride or pile a few extra plates on the barbell—and you should learn to take advantage of those, too.

Though the programs in this book are designed for maximum effectiveness *and* safety, you should still monitor yourself, play it safe when you have to, and amp it up when you're feeling turbocharged. It'll keep you in the game that much longer.

7. Thou Shalt Be Social.

This one can be a matter of taste: Some people are lone-wolf exercisers; others can barely bring themselves to step out the door without a platoon of fellow runners urging them onward. Generally I'd suggest you figure out which way works for you and stick with it most of the time.

I will say this, however, to inveterate solo exercisers: Working out with others is a whole new ball game. Competitive types will find that having other people around automatically raises the stakes on their workouts, and will take each set, rep, and lap more seriously. Social types will look forward to catching up with friends, and will be more consistent in their workouts because they're accountable to them. And every adult, male or female, should reexperience the joys of being part of a team once in a while—in a rec or league sport, for instance, or on a mud run or adventure race. Forget the traumas of gym class: Teamwork solidifies and deepens friendships while giving you added motivation to work hard and do your best.

8. Thou Shalt Fuel Thy Body Well.

You hear it from fitness pros all the time: *You can't out-train a bad diet.* The math is fairly straightforward: Hit the gym hard for an hour or so and you might burn 500 calories. But if you stop at Starbucks on the way home and grab a scone and a white-chocolate mocha, you could easily down *700 calories* without a second thought. *Working out doesn't give you a license to gorge.*

The good news is that regular exercisers gravitate toward better eating as a matter of course. Maybe it's their bodies telling them what they need; maybe it's the little shot of willpower that regular working out affords them. Regardless, if you need to clean up your diet, there's no better time to do it than when you're embarking on a new exercise program—you'll look and feel better, and you'll get even better results from your new program.

So, what constitutes good fuel? I like to keep it simple: Part 4 of this book is all you'll ever need to know about eating and diet. Heck, rip out those pages, frame them, and hang them on your wall. These few principles will help you lose weight, build and maintain muscle mass, and feel great for a lifetime.

Best of all, you won't have to change eating strategies every time a new diet title goes soaring up the bestseller charts. It's advice that will never go out of style.

9. Thou Shalt Rest. Exercise
and nutrition are only part of the weight-loss and fitness equation. The other major component—which can easily make or break an exercise program—is rest.

Adequate rest stimulates the *parasympathetic nervous system*—a cascade of physical and psychological responses that calm you down and set the stage for fat burning, muscle growth, good digestion, and cell repair. This system counterbalances the *sympathetic nervous system,* the heart-pounding, sweat-dripping, "freeze, flight or fight" response stimulated by various types of stress—including vigorous exercise.

Stress gets a bad name in our culture, but it's only really a problem when it's unrelieved by periods of rest and recuperation. Without adequate rest to balance out the stresses in your life, your body gets stuck in a continuous game of catch-up ball, never quite able to undo the damage you're inflicting. Illness, injury, and chronic fatigue can result.

Eight hours of sleep a night is standard—some need more, and a few need a little less. If you're consistently getting *much* less, you're definitely not operating at full capacity, however. Find ways to get more, either by napping or powering down earlier in the evening, and you'll be surprised at how alert and productive you can be during the day. And how little caffeine you need to get by.

You should also take scheduled time off from intense exercise. I recommend doing some form of exercise every day of the week, but a couple of days should be reserved for active rest. Pilates or yoga are a great choice on these days—they enhance mobility, flexibility, and core strength without overstressing your joints or muscles. Light aerobic exercise like walking, easy biking, or jogging for fitter exercisers can also alleviate soreness, speed recovery from stress, and help you unwind before bedtime.

10. Thou Shalt Minimize Sitting.

You probably think of sitting as a neutral activity: Something that doesn't do you much good but can't do you much harm, either. Unfortunately, that's not the case. Recent research suggests that sitting for 11 hours a day or more increases your chances of dying from any cause by a stunning 40 percent—and that's independent of all other factors, including age, education, and physical activity. So the half-hour jog you squeeze in on your lunch break, while beneficial, doesn't fully offset the many more hours you spend at your desk, on the couch, and behind the wheel. String together enough years of sitting on your butt for both work and pleasure, and your body more or less forgets how to do much else.

How to avoid this fate? Simple: Move. As much as possible, as often as possible.

The consensus on this is that for every 20 minutes you spend at your desk, you should spend 2 minutes standing, walking, or stretching. Once you establish the habit, it will improve your productivity, sharpen your focus, and help you think more clearly.

BONUS COMMANDMENT: Thou Shalt Not Be Perfect.

One major obstacle people struggle with in their quest for fitness is perfectionism: They think that if they can't do an hour-long workout in their local gym with its spandexed denizens and gleaming chrome dumbbells, topped off by a steam bath and a massage, they might as well do nothing at all. They compare themselves to athletes and airbrushed movie stars and think they'll never measure up, believing that if they aren't sporting a twelve-pack or wearing a size zero dress, they're a failure in the fitness department. They miss a workout and think they've irrevocably blown it.

Folks, it ain't so. Studies have shown substantial benefits from just *10 minutes* of daily exercise, and these days, smart trainers have figured out ways to cram serious training sessions into that amount of time or less. So forget the time-constraint worry. Do whatever you can fit in on the days when you're overcommitted, and resolve to fit in a little more on your next serious workout day.

Further studies have indicated that when obese people raise their fitness level, they substantially lower their risk of heart disease *even if they don't lose a pound*. So while seeing external changes—and looking a little more like those retouched media images—can be motivating, understand that the changes you can't see may be even more important to your health and longevity. And those changes can come very quickly.

Give yourself permission to fail, to look awkward, to be a rank beginner. Babies and toddlers learn new physical skills at an astounding rate. You know why?

They aren't afraid to stink at something.

SECRETS OF THE "REAL" BIGGEST LOSERS

The *Biggest Loser* crowd has their methods: injury-inducing workouts, tyrannical trainers who berate and belittle, public humiliation on a nationwide scale. Makes for great ratings—but, as numerous follow-up stories have shown, not the most successful losers. Not in the long term, anyway.

So who are real biggest losers? Are there any out there?

Turns out there are—and they're helping us understand successful weight loss away from the camera glare of reality TV. The National Weight Control Registry was established in 1994 to track the behavior and results of people who have lost substantial amounts of weight and kept it off for long periods. To date, their research includes data from over 10,000 individuals who have lost an average of 66 pounds and kept it off for an average of 5.5 years.

Instead of dramatic, sweat-pouring workouts, most of these people simply make a hundred small decisions a day that add up to extraordinary results.

Some of their findings:

• Some of the members lost weight quickly, while others did so over as many as 14 years.

• 45 percent of the members lost weight on their own; the other 55 percent lost weight with the help of some type of program.

• 98 percent modified their food intake in some way, with most reporting that they follow a low-calorie, low-fat diet.

• 94 percent increased physical activity in some way, with the most common activity being walking.

• 78 percent eat breakfast every day.

• 75 percent weigh themselves at least once a week.

• 62 percent watch less than 10 hours of TV per week.

• 90 percent exercise an average of 1 hour per day.

Nothing too dramatic or camera worthy: just a lot of common sense, applied scrupulously over long periods of time. Says one registry member, "I'm just an ordinary person. But I do a whole bunch of very, very tiny things every day that *together* are extraordinary."

How Much Exercise? The Minimum Effective Dose

When treating patients, doctors work with the principle of the "minimum effective dose": When prescribing medication, we're taught to ask, what's the least amount we can give the patient and still see the results we're looking for?

In a medical context, this makes perfect sense: Many medications come with undesirable side effects that are best kept at a minimum. And as doctors, we never want to impede the sometimes-mysterious workings of the human immune system. So to us, the minimum effective dose concept works beautifully. As the saying goes, "First, do no harm."

So if exercise is medicine, what amount will give you the maximum health benefit for the least amount of time and energy invested? Is there a minimum effective dose?

I believe that there is.

Exercise differs from most medications in that more if it is almost *always* better. The side effects of exercise—weight loss, preservation of muscle mass, greater longevity, improved mood, better-functioning body systems, and so on—are all beneficial. And they tend to increase with the more "medicine" you take.

I can't think of another medication where that's the case.

So what's the quantity of exercise—the dosage—where we can feel confident we've derived *most*, if not all, of its benefits? The science is pretty clear: The major health benefits of exercise appear to level off at around 150 minutes a week. That amounts to about a half hour of exercise, 5 days a week, of brisk walking. Do something more intense—say, jogging—and that counts double. In the 1990s, a study of 8,000 employees at the Osaka gas company in Japan found that, among employees who walked to work, those whose walk took more than 20 minutes had a 30 percent lower chance of getting hypertension: A tiny investment of time for such a massive payoff. Every 10-minute increase in the duration of their walk to work netted them a 12 percent drop in their chances of developing this chronic, dangerous condition.

Believe it or not, that's it. If, right now, you're completely sedentary and start doing *just that much*, your risk of heart disease drops. Your insulin sensitivity and your HDL, or good cholesterol levels, go up while your serum triglycerides, blood pressure, and your chances of obesity go down. Stress dissipates. Focus and productivity improve. You'll play better with others.

The beauty of being a complete beginner is that you get more benefit out of your exercise program than virtually anyone else. If I added another workout to my schedule, or one of my pro athlete patients tried to sneak in another session in the weight room or on the track next week, they'd get very little health benefit out of it. They might even get injured and make themselves less healthy. But a beginner is different. To a beginner, 150 minutes in a week is life changing.

There's a final benefit to exercising regularly that isn't even covered in the literature. Exercise 150 minutes a week for 3 weeks, without fail, and you'll have established a habit of self-care that will serve you in good stead for the rest of your life. If you build that half hour into your day for exercise most days of the week, you may eventually have the overwhelming urge to add to it: Make it an hour, make it not a walk but a run or a swim or a bike ride or a game of Ultimate Frisbee. And at that point, the health benefits start to compound.

"What If I Want More?"

As powerful and effective as 150 minutes per week can be, they will *not* get you to maximum performance. You won't be dunking any basketballs, running any marathons, or sporting a head-turning physique by taking a few walks a week. To achieve goals like those, you'll have to put in a little more.

One of the reasons that recommended parameters for physical activity and fitness change so much is that there's no clear definition of being fit. You first have to answer the question, "Fit for what?" Even an

unfit person is fit for something, after all: They're fit for the unchallenging demands they've been placing on their bodies. Just as a high level of physical fitness is an adaptation, so is low fitness simply your body's way of adapting to the demands you're placing—or not placing—on it.

If you want to complete an endurance race or show off a set of six-pack abs, you've got to train for those specific goals. A simple low-impact exercise routine won't get you there. Daily walking *will* improve your health enormously, lower your chances of contracting many serious illnesses, lift your mood, and make your doctor weep with joy.

If, however, you decide you want more out of your fitness program— more fitness, more strength, more glowing health—you'll need to put more into it. How to do that is the focus of this section of the book.

Choose Your Level

All told, there are 9 months of structured workouts in the pages that follow—plus a few side detours here and there—that break neatly into three 3-month chunks. A beginner can do all 9 months sequentially— repeating a phase if necessary; others may want to start later in the program.

You can also self-manage the time frames. Work a plan for

4 weeks, for example, then pause to evaluate your progress. Maybe you'll want to change up your routine. Do it! The goal is regular exercise and fun.

Here's how to determine your readiness for each level:

BRONZE (BEGINNER) LEVEL:

You're either a complete beginner or you're coming back from a long enough layoff so you feel like one. Maybe it's an injury or illness, but for whatever reason, you've been away from exercise and it's time to get back on the horse.

SILVER (INTERMEDIATE) LEVEL:
You exercise, but it's been sporadic. You know a lot of what the gym has to offer, and maybe a couple of sports as well. Maybe you've lost your way, lost interest, need a boost and some new ideas. Here's where

you start: challenging, but not too intimidating.

GOLD (ADVANCED) LEVEL:
You're one of the faithful. You don't miss many workouts, and when you do, it's not a good day—for you or anyone who crosses your path. You might play a sport or two regularly, or compete in endurance events, in addition to staying diligent with your exercise program. This is the program you want to get to the next level of mastery.

Let's Get Ready to Rumble!

Okay, you've read all about the benefits of exercise. You've read about how to assess your fitness level and where you should start.

Now? Time to start!

Can You OD on the World's Most Effective Medicine? Yes!

Is there a point where additional exercise ceases to be beneficial? Yes. Exercise physiologists call it "overtraining syndrome," a condition of chronic exhaustion that occurs after many months, and sometimes years, of regular, intense exercise.

The term "overtraining" gets tossed around a little too casually for my taste by weekend warrior types: They'll get a little more sore than usual, claim to be overtrained, and use it as an excuse to skip out on exercise altogether for weeks at a time. And, of course, endurance athletes who are serious about their sport (myself included!) are inaccurately called "exercise addicts" all the time. The last thing I want to do in this book is to scare anyone away from of working up a serious sweat on a regular basis.

To clarify: True "overtraining syndrome" is *not* simply a matter of going at it too hard in a workout or two. According to Abby Ruby, PhD, author of *In Sickness and in Health: Exercise Addiction in Endurance Athletes,* "Most often what appears to be overtraining is simply under-fueling or under-recovering." In the average athletic career, you're much more likely to "overreach" a bit—work a little too hard in one or two workouts—than you are to truly overtrain. Given adequate sleep and good food, you should recover from an overreach in a few days.

Similarly, there's a fundamental difference between being a disciplined exerciser—even training many hours a day, in some cases—and being an "exercise addict." If there weren't such a difference, every pro athlete in the world would be considered pathological. But they aren't: They're just people like you and me, driven to do a good job at their chosen profession of athletics.

Here are the primary symptoms, both physical and psychological:

• **Physical:** The number-one red flag: You've stopped improving. No matter how many more miles or hours or reps you put in, you can't get any faster, stronger, or better. Your body has stopped responding to exercise and the plateau has gone on for several months.

Also, most people who overtrain will eventually incur "high-risk" overuse injuries. Examples include stress fractures around the hip and high-grade partial tears of tendons from repetitive use. Athletes who suffer these high-risk overuse injuries have inevitably disregarded their body's pain cues and made their injuries much worse. Characteristically, they push and push and the injuries go from bad to terrible, often taking many months to heal.

Typically, the physical manifestations of overtraining eventually wind up sidelining the athlete completely—at which point he or she is forced to confront the condition head-on.

• **Psychological:** In most cases, the exercise addict no longer enjoys exercise: They tend to treat every training session like their worst day at work, and if they compete, they dread their races. These athletes aren't just nervous: They're exhausted and look it.

Addicts continue to train through (though not *around)*

pain and injury, and will exercise despite illness, negative effects on relationships, jobs, finances, and other red flags that it's time to back off. They're unable to take days off from training. When they miss a workout, anxiety skyrockets. Sometimes, people fall into overtraining when they're trying to deal with—or perhaps more accurately, *avoid* dealing with—a death, divorce, job loss, or other life trauma.

Although the physical symptoms of overtraining are strong indications of a problem, it's ultimately this *attitude* toward exercise—in which working out takes priority over virtually everything else—that defines addiction.

BRONZE

THE BEGINNER PROGRAM:
MONTHS 1–3

You haven't so much as laced on your training shoes since middle-school gym class. You have an aversion to walking—much less climbing stairs, jogging, or going to an actual gym. Or you might be a chronic restarter: You work out hard for a couple of weeks, and maybe even start to see and feel some results. But then life interferes again, your schedule gets tight, and you miss a workout. Rather than forgive yourself, you throw up your hands and fall out of the habit. Or maybe you're coming back after an exercise layoff after an illness, injury, or other life-changing event that took you out of the game for 6 months or more. Regardless of your circumstances, you've decided to give exercise a try.

That's great news! Here's some more: Everything you need to start is right here.

BRONZE
MONTH 1
THE FIRST
WORKOUT

First off: congratulations. As in most endeavors, the first step in starting an exercise program is the toughest—especially if you've tried to commit to regular exercise in the past and your efforts have fallen short. So you're to be commended for taking it this far: A 2010 survey found that only about half of all Americans exercise even 3 days a week—and a depressing 5 percent get regular vigorous exercise. So that's why you already have a bronze medal in my book—you're already running ahead of 95 percent of the population.

I sincerely want you to succeed, and so these first few weeks on a program are going to be crucial. I want you to establish the habit, to carve out the time you need to exercise consistently and well. The habit begins when you decide that your health is actually worth taking time for. Once you've made that leap, the sky's the limit.

So in a way, at first, it almost doesn't matter *what* you do, just that you set aside time to do *something*.

Almost—but not quite. I am going to give you an actual workout program.

Here it is: The first month, all I want you to do is to walk for a half hour every day. That's it. That's your workout: *the minimum effective dose that I wrote about in the last section.*

Why so little? Why don't I recommend *more*, when enthusiasm is *high* and you're raring to go?

Here's why: Most people start an exercise program with the best of intentions. Brimming with enthusiasm and determination to meet a new fitness goal ("Get in shape by summertime!" "Lose three dress sizes by St. Patty's!" or my favorite, "Train for a marathon in 6 weeks!"), they attack their workouts with vigor—and burn out after a few days.

You've got to trust me on this. I don't care if you're a former champion triathlete or a power lifter with nine state championships to your name. If you've been away from exercise for 6 months or more, your assignment is so simple, I'm just going to say it again:

Walk for a half hour a day every day for a month.

If you're familiar with Zen, or more likely *The Karate Kid*, this first month is the equivalent of the scene when the new student visits the master and asks to be taught his secrets. He's ready for anything, ready to dive in and *work*, ready to prove his strength and manliness and commitment.

But the master assigns him menial tasks that appear to have nothing to do with what the student asked to learn. Day after day, the student returns, and day after day, the master has him do menial tasks: chopping wood, carrying water. Painting the fence, sanding the floor. Wax on, wax off.

The student grows impatient. Frustrated. He wants to give up. But then, at some point, he realizes that the key to the art he wanted to learn is actually implanted in the mundane tasks the master has asked him to do.

In this case, it's the gospel truth. If you've read the book so far, you know that many of the benefits of exercise that I've spent all these pages describing can be derived from this simple workout. People who go from no exercise to a half-hour daily walk experience health changes that are literally transformative, much more so than the already-dedicated exerciser who ratchets up the intensity on workouts that are already far beyond what's needed for good health. At that stage, you're really just tweaking.

By contrast, going from *no* exercise a week to a total of over *200 minutes* a week as this simple program suggests will give you untold health benefits that you can't imagine. So much so that if this is all you do—if you never progress past this beginning stage—you'll still rack up the benefits:

• Your cardiovascular health will improve.

• Your bone density will increase, particularly in your legs.

• Your muscles and connective tissue will strengthen and grow.

• Your outlook, mood, and ability to focus will improve.

You don't even have to do all 30 minutes at once: Ten minutes in the morning, 10 in the afternoon, 10 before bed is fine, though I think it's advisable, given what's to come, to do the whole thing at once. The later workouts in this program are harder to do in this broken-up way, so you might want to prep for them by doing all your walking at once. You may also find it easier to just get it out of the way.

So: This month, walk. Establish the habit. Don't weigh yourself, snap photos, or even look ahead to see what's to come. Take your walks, enjoy them, and *then* turn the page.

Remember, an exercise habit is a marathon, not a sprint. You're going to be doing this for a long time. There's plenty of time for sweat, intensity, and mayhem in the coming weeks.

See you next month.

GET EVEN BETTER RESULTS:
Become a "NEAT" Freak

As you take on your workouts this month, I want you to work on your NEAT-ness. But I'm not talking about your closets or your desk drawer: I'm talking about finding ways to sit less.

"Sitting," says Dr. James Levine, an endocrinologist at the Mayo Clinic who has researched the dangers of a sedentary life for the last 15 years, "is the new smoking." Levine's studies have shown that sitting around—as many of us do for both work *and* pleasure—is bad for your health. Spending more than just 6 hours a day on your backside drives up blood pressure and places you at a greater risk for diabetes, obesity, depression, and some types of cancer. People who already have chronic illnesses see an increase in their symptoms. And that's just for starters.

Think you're out of danger if you go to the gym regularly? Think again: The usual guidelines for regular exercise simply aren't enough to counteract the dangers of all the sitting we do. And we do a lot of it: Americans average 9.5 hours on our collective butts per day. That's a lot of smoking.

So maybe it's possible to limit our time on the couch. But when you make your living sitting at a desk, what's to be done?

The answer is NEAT—*nonexercise activity thermogenesis*. In other words, getting up and moving around, at an easy pace, as often as possible, for as long as possible. NEAT used to be far

more interwoven into our lives: Walk to the post office. Walk down the hall to confer with a coworker. Walk to the market and walk back with the groceries. These days? Not so much: Technology allows us to do almost everything from the comfort of a chair.

This may help to explain why we're getting so much heavier than the Americans just a few generations back, even as we have become more and more obsessed with fitness. Our grandparents certainly didn't have a big-box gym on every corner. As a group, in fact, people probably got less formal exercise than we get today. Without the conveniences of e-mail and other labor-saving technologies, day-to-day lives simply required more movement 50 or 100 years ago. And since even slow walking can more than double your metabolic rate compared with sitting, you can see how being just a little more active during your day can make a huge difference to your weight and health.

Still don't think walking "counts" as exercise? A 2004 study of the Amish—a modern agrarian culture that shuns post–industrial revolution technology—indicates that as a group, they're remarkably healthy: Cancer rates are far lower than those of the country at large, and obesity is almost nonexistent, despite a conspicuous lack of treadmills and weights in their communities, and a diet rich in meat, pie, refined sugar, and other fattening foods. Their apparent secret? High amounts of NEAT: Amish women take about 14,000 steps a day, and Amish men are up around 18,000—something on the order of 8 miles a day.

I'm not suggesting we dispense with all technology and live like the Amish. But I am saying we need to figure out ways to make our own NEAT. You've may have heard this fitness tidbit before and dismissed it as impractical. Who has time for all that walking?

The surprising answer: You do. Even if you don't want to spring for a treadmill-desk (they do exist!), there are lots of ways to sneak more easy, focus-building, nonsweaty NEAT into your life. Here are a few:

1. Walk and Talk. As a culture, we conduct most of our business and social affairs from a seated position: in restaurants, boardrooms, and coffee shops. Whenever possible, find ways to turn these into walking meetings—especially when you're meeting one-on-one: Offer to stroll in the park or around the block rather than sitting down and eating something you probably don't need. You'll eat less, move more, and probably even think better: Walking can help your ideas flow.

2. Go Mobile. Many of us who grew up with desktops and wall phones are still stuck to the idea that *we* have to be stuck while using mobile devices like cell phones and laptops. So we sit at a desk while chatting on our cell phone or working away on a laptop. Whenever you're on the phone, take it as an opportunity to walk—or at least stand. Most people feel—and sound—more engaged when they're on their feet, so you'll make a better impression on the phone if you're up and about anyway. And change locations with your laptop whenever possible: Take it to a park, a café, another room in your house.

3. Take a Microbreak. One of the reasons it's so tough to maintain good posture at a desk is that your ligaments and other soft tissues start to deform after about 20 minutes in the same position, gradually giving your body a permanently chair-shaped appearance. Fight this tendency with 1- to 5-minute breaks for every 20 minutes you're at work: Stretch, breathe, focus your eyes on a distant object. You'll come back to work refreshed and recommitted.

4. Steal a Workout. This falls under the no-brainer category: Grab the first parking spot you see in the lot (the farther away from the door, the better) rather than circling for 10 minutes looking for the perfect one. Take the stairs, not the elevator. And stay off the human conveyor belt at the airport, too: You're going to be stuck on a plane for 6 hours anyway—do you really need *less* activity? Whenever there's a choice—walk. This may seem like novice advice, but it can make a huge difference in the number of calories you burn in a given day.

5. Miss your stop . . . on Purpose. If you use public transportation, try getting off a stop before or a stop after the one most convenient to your destination. You'll be able to squeeze in 10 or 15 minutes of pleasant walking—and maybe get to know your neighborhood a little better at the same time.

6. Go for Face Time (not the app). I'm lucky that my profession requires me to see people face-to-face: It's hard to diagnose a torn meniscus or a separated shoulder over e-mail. But many people can go through their workday without ever actually interacting with their closest coworkers. They text the guy down the hall, they e-mail blast to their most valuable clients. Nothing wrong with convenience. But if you've got a question for Linda, and she's right down the hall, take the 3-minute break and go see her. Chances are you'll communicate better anyway.

7. Get Less Efficient. In the movie *Wall-E*, the people of the future live on Barc-o-lounger-shaped scooter-chairs that zip them from place to place, dispensing a never-ending stream of soft drinks into their big-gulp-size cups. It's not too far off from where we appear to be headed right now. Efficiency, it seems, is killing us. One novel solution is to get a little inefficient on purpose: Set up your work station so you have to reach for things rather than keeping them within an arm's reach. Put the file cabinet and wastebasket a ways away so you *have* to walk over to them (or at least practice your free throw). Reaching, stretching, extending,

and of course, walking feel great, especially when you've been stuck in the chair all morning.

8. Leverage Your TV Time. I personally don't know anyone who admits to watching more than an hour of television a day—but with the national average up around 5 hours, I know they're out there. TV time can be invaluable for stretching, floor Pilates, and yoga postures. No need to make it superintense: Restorative postures are great, especially if you're winding down before bed. You'll sleep better, burn a few calories, and shave some time off your sitting hours for the day. And you'll relieve a little of the guilt from your favorite guilty pleasure.

9. Include the Family. This applies to any fitness venture: a better diet, a more stringent workout program, a more active lifestyle. Don't go it alone. Make sure everyone near you—especially your family—knows that you're trying to get more activity into your day, and include them as much as you can in the effort. Take a walk around the block instead of a trip to get fast food; play mini-golf instead of going to the movies; choose Twister instead of video games. It's okay if you're not a superathletic family—you don't have to shoot hoops and shag fly balls every night. But the more *incidentally* active your family activities can be, the better. And you'll be instilling the importance of regular movement into your kids' lives—and that's a pretty important gift.

CHANGE YOUR BEHAVIOR, CHANGE YOUR LIFE

There's a huge difference between *knowing* something and *doing* it.

Obesity rates in the United States—currently 36 percent of adults and 17 percent of children—have risen dramatically in the last decade. Junk food sales have climbed steadily in that time: From the 1950s to the early 2000s, consumption of sweeteners of all kinds went up 39 percent in the United States; in that same time frame, our consumption of corn sweeteners *octupled*. Screen time in the United States is up at around 5.5 hours. Among minorities, it's closer to 8 hours.

All this in a country that spent about $61 billion on weight-loss products and information in 2010—up from $59 billion in 2008.

The point: We don't lack for information. What we lack for is the "hows" of behavior change, the day-to-day strategies that we can implement to help us stop old behaviors and implement new ones.

So how do you effect real change in your behavior?

Ease into it. Start with a small step that's easy and fun. Change one small, easy thing today, another one next week, and so on.

Make those changes small and specific: Eat an apple instead of a candy bar for your midmorning snack. Switch to water instead of soda for lunch. Take the stairs up to your office in the morning. Be meticulous about your planning—preparing not just what you're going to do but how you're going to do it. If you decide that you're going to eat three pieces of fruit every day, for example, that means you need to buy 21 pieces of fruit. When

and where are you going to get them? What kinds of fruit are you going to get? Where are you going to store them? Are you going to eat them for breakfast, lunch, dinner, or all three?

These seem like tiny details, but they're essential. They make the difference between fitness as an abstract idea and a concrete, workable plan. Know the where-who-why-how of your plan, not just the broad strokes, and you'll be that much more likely to implement it.

You'll see some of these strategies detailed throughout this book. But the most effective ones for you will be based on the specifics of your life. Getting up early to work out won't work for the night-shifter, and eating grass-fed beef won't work for the vegetarian.

In general, though, choose the actions you feel you can maintain—even when life gets stressful and temptation rears its head. The fancy gym on the other side of town may seem appealing, but will you still be willing to make the trek when work stress goes through the roof? Or would you be better off choosing the less-fancy but acceptable gym that's walking distance from work? If you're going out to eat, are you going to be able to choose the grilled chicken if you go to your favorite burger joint, or would it be better to go somewhere healthy where temptation isn't just a few feet away, sizzling on the grill?

Only you can answer those questions for yourself, but I suggest you choose according to what makes the successful, healthy choice the easiest one to make.

If you followed the directions in the previous section, you've now, officially, established an exercise habit. Well done. Maybe it was easier than you thought—but maybe not. The point of month 1 was to get you moving regularly and, ideally, to make you hungry for more.

This section is all about that something more. In this second month, I'm going to introduce two new ideas—foam rolling and mobility work—my version of warming up, which in this program takes the form of *dynamic stretching*. These two new elements are going to raise the technical bar on what you've been doing significantly: Yup, now we're talking real exercises that you'll have to learn.

Don't let that throw you. Learning is an essential part of an exercise program, and the first stage of learning is doing something that at first feels awkward and unfamiliar. So if you find yourself feeling klutzy in this second month, that's actually a very good sign: You're forcing your body to adapt and change. Let yourself learn. Your brain was made for it.

You're also going to continue your walking routine, a half hour daily, but now I want to add something to the mix: tracking your heart rate.

The Secret to Big Training Gains

Triathletes and marathoners live by the strength and endurance of their heart muscles. They brag about the glacial rate of their heart's beat at rest; they'll tie themselves in rhetorical knots trying to work their VO2-max score into casual conversation whenever possible; they'll wear heart rate monitors all day long and track their progress by the minutest shifts in the pounding of their ever-toiling tickers.

You don't need to go that far. You're still a beginner.

For now, here's all I want you to do. Carry a timepiece with a second hand when you walk. A stopwatch works, too. Every 10 minutes or so, starting 5 minutes into your walk, pull out your watch and take your pulse at your carotid artery (lift your chin, place the tips of your index and second fingers to one side of your windpipe, and count away—your pulse should be clear as a bell). Keep track of the pulse for 6 seconds.

There are several formulas for calculating your ideal heart rate during aerobic exercise. Some seem to require several years of higher math to understand. I'm going to keep it simple for you. Check the following chart—it shows age to the left, beats per 6-second interval to the right:

HEART RATE FOR AEROBIC EXERCISE

AGE	BEATS IN 6 SECONDS
30s	11–13
40s	10–12
50s	10–12
60s	9–11
70s	9–10
80s	8–9

So if you're 55 years old, you want your pulse reading to be anywhere from 10 to 12 beats in 6 seconds. That comes out to 100 to 120 beats a minute, which, for a 55-year-old, comes out to anywhere from 60 to 70 percent of your maximum heart rate.

Don't be too concerned about maximum heart rate percentages for now: From experience, I know plenty of people who fall way outside that range, on both the low and the high side. That's why what we're looking for here is a ballpark.

So: What to do if your heart rate is too low? Walk faster. Walk up a hill. Take it into an easy jog if you feel so inclined. Just work a little harder and check it again in 10 minutes. If you get uncomfortable working at this tougher intensity, back off a little (don't stop!) until you're ready to go at it again. Over the course of the month, work up to keeping your heart rate in that zone for the full 30 minutes.

What if it's too high? The standard advice is to back off, but I disagree—as long as you're *comfortable* exercising at the higher rate. If you aren't, slow down a bit. But if you feel fine, keep it up. Some people are very comfortable exercising at faster heart rates for long periods, and I wouldn't want to hold you back!

In addition to your walking, I want you to do two other routines: foam rolling and dynamic stretching, at least three times a week each. Feel free to do them more often—neither is very difficult, and both feel great once you're used to them. Each routine will take you less than 10 minutes, so you'll only be adding a total of an hour of workout time to your entire week. Scheduling-wise, your workout week might look like this:

YOUR BRONZE MONTH 2 ROUTINE

MONDAY:	Foam rolling, walk
TUESDAY:	Dynamic stretch #1, walk
WEDNESDAY:	Foam rolling, walk
THURSDAY:	Walk only
FRIDAY:	Dynamic stretch #2, walk
SATURDAY:	Foam rolling, walk
SUNDAY:	Dynamic stretch #1, walk

VARIATIONS:

If you want to mix up this regimen, you can. There are two dynamic stretching routines, which you can alternate between or switch between as the mood grabs you: The next week you might do the second dynamic stretch routine twice and the first one only once.

You can put the "walk-only" day on any day of the week—just pick up where you left off on the foam rolling and dynamic stretching routines after that day. I'd also suggest that you consider making your "walk-only" day slightly longer, more challenging, or in a new and different place than usual. If you take a short hike with your family or friends over the weekend, make that your longer walk. You've got 10 more minutes than usual on that day: Use 'em.

The Workouts: Foam Rolling

If you only buy one piece of exercise equipment for the rest of your life, make it a foam roller. It's so simple and so brilliant. The foam roller is a piece of dense, industrial-grade Styrofoam. It's also the most convenient, reliable, and inexpensive massage therapist money can buy.

By positioning yourself on the roller and oscillating back and forth over your muscles and connective tissues in various ways, you can give yourself a deep and effective massage for virtually any part of your body.

Once you learn how to do it, a full foam-rolling routine lasts only a few minutes, and you'll notice immediate changes in your ease of move-

ment, posture, and mobility. Without stretching at all, you'll feel looser and more flexible—as if you've developed a healthier body almost instantaneously.

How can this be? By squeezing, pushing, and kneading your major muscles, foam rolling directly affects the suppleness of your *fascia*—the white, pliable, mesh-like substance that goes through and around all your muscles. Fascia is highly adaptable. It supports and reinforces any physical habit you have, good or bad. All the sitting most of us do, for example, is written in the fascia. If you could peel back the skin of a chronic desk-sitter, the fascia would probably be thick and tight around the hip joints and midback. Right-handed tennis players and golfers have visible asymmetries in their fascial systems as well.

Adhesions in the fascial web resemble knots in a bungee cord, inhibiting its ability to extend fully. A knotted cord still stretches, of course—it just stretches a whole lot better if you get the knots out first. Over time, foam rolling will do that for you.

After you get the hang of this routine, it will take you less than 10 minutes and leave you feeling fantastic.

Fair warning: Like a deep massage, foam rolling can be uncomfortable. At first. Typically, your most tender areas are the places that need it the most—but over time, you'll become less sensitive, a sign that you're effectively smoothing out those fascial knots.

THE FOAM-ROLLING ROUTINE

Perform the following movements at least three times a week before your workouts—more often if you can. Spend about 30 seconds on each muscle group—more if they are particularly tender.

HAMSTRING ROLL

• Place a foam roller under your right knee, with your leg straight. Cross your left leg over your right ankle. Put your hands flat on the floor for support. Keep your back naturally arched.

• Roll your body forward until the roller reaches your glutes. Then roll back and forth. Repeat with the roller under your left thigh.

NOTE: If rolling one leg is too difficult, perform the movement with both legs on the roller.

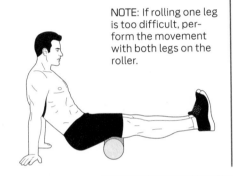

GLUTE ROLL

• Sit with a foam roller positioned on the back of your right thigh, just below your glutes. Cross your right leg over the front of your left thigh. Put your hands flat on the floor for support.

• Roll your body forward until the roller reaches your lower back. Then roll back and forth. Repeat with the roller under your left glute.

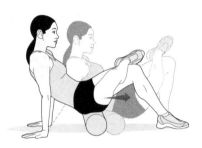

ILIOTIBIAL-BAND ROLL

• Lie on your right side and place your right hip on a foam roller. Put your right forearm on the floor for support. Cross your left leg over your right and place your left foot flat on the floor.

• Roll your body forward until the roller reaches your knee. Then roll back and forth. Lie on your left side and repeat with the roller under your left hip. (If this becomes too easy over time, place your left leg on top of your right instead of bracing it on the floor.)

IMPORTANT NOTE: Your iliotibial band—commonly called the IT band—is a tough strip of connective tissue that runs down the side of your thigh, starting on your hip bone and connecting just below your knee. When you start foam rolling, you'll probably find that this tissue is one of the most sensitive areas that you can roll over, perhaps due to the high tension of the band. Remember, pain means you need to roll it. Make this a priority, because over time, if your IT band is too tight, it could cause knee pain.

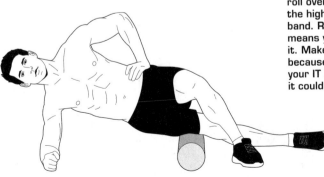

THE FOAM-ROLLING ROUTINE—*Continued*

CALF ROLL
• Place a foam roller under your right ankle, with your right leg straight. Cross your left leg over your right ankle. Put your hands flat on the floor for support and keep your back naturally arched.

• Roll your body forward until the roller reaches the back of your right knee. Then roll back and forth. Repeat with the roller under your left calf. (If this is too hard, perform the movement with both legs on the roller.)

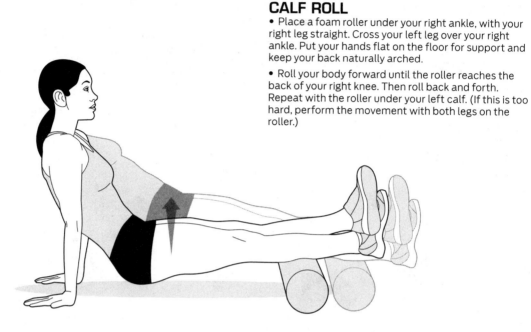

QUADRICEPS-AND-HIP-FLEXOR ROLL
• Lie facedown on the floor with a foam roller positioned above your right knee. Cross your left leg over your right ankle and place your elbows on the floor for support.

• Roll your body backward until the roller reaches the top of your right thigh. Then roll back and forth. Repeat with the roller under your left thigh. (If that's too hard, perform the movement with both thighs on the roller.)

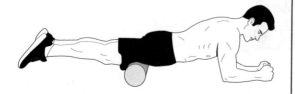

GROIN ROLL
• Lie facedown on the floor. Place a foam roller parallel to your body. Put your elbows on the floor for support. Position your right thigh nearly perpendicular to your body, with the inner portion of your thigh, just above the level of your knee, resting on top of the roller.

• Roll your body toward the right until the roller reaches your pelvis. Then roll back and forth. Repeat with the roller under your left thigh.

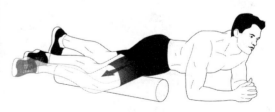

LOWER-BACK ROLL

Lie faceup with a foam roller under your midback. Your knees should be bent, with your feet flat on the floor. Raise your hips off the floor slightly. Roll back and forth over your lower back.

UPPER-BACK ROLL

• Lie faceup with a foam roller under your midback, at the bottom of your shoulder blades. Clasp your hands behind your head and pull your elbows toward each other. Raise your hips off the floor slightly.

• Slowly lower your back downward, so that your upper back bends over the foam roller. Raise back to the start and roll forward a couple of inches—so that the roller sits higher under your upper back—and repeat. Roll forward one more time and do it again. That's 1 rep.

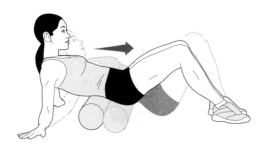
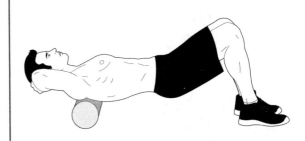

SHOULDER-BLADE ROLL

• Lie faceup with a foam roller under your upper back, at the tops of your shoulder blades. Cross your arms over your chest. Your knees should be bent with your feet flat on the floor.

• Raise your hips so they're slightly elevated off the floor. Roll back and forth over your shoulder blades and your mid- and upper back.

BONUS ROLL: THE FEET

A foam roller is too big for your feet, but rolling a tennis ball back-and-forth under your foot is a great way to keep the plantar fascia (the tight band running on the underside of each foot) supple. It's also a great way to help prevent plantar fasciitis, a painful and debilitating strain of that tissue.

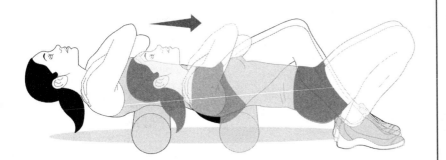

DYNAMIC STRETCHING AND WARMUP:
THE NEW-OLD KID ON THE BLOCK

If you're a dedicated stretcher, you may be surprised to learn that standard, reach-and-hold flexibility exercises before a workout aren't necessarily a great idea. Numerous studies have shown that those types of moves actually reduce your strength and power temporarily. More effective in prepping you for a tough workout is dynamic stretching, moves that look very similar to old-school calisthenics.

Turns out that all those turn-of-the-century, bloomer-wearing gymnasium types were on to something. Swinging your limbs, kicking, and jumping in ways that put your joints through a large, athletic range of motion prime your body for a workout much better than slower, more meditative stretches. Following are a few of the best, divided into two routines, which you can alternate at will.

DYNAMIC STRETCHING: ROUTINE #1
This warmup is simple. Do 10 reps of each of these exercises with no rest between sets:

JUMPING JACK
Stand with your feet together and your hands at your sides. Simultaneously raise your arms above your head and jump up just enough to spread your feet out wide. Without pause, quickly reverse the movement and repeat.

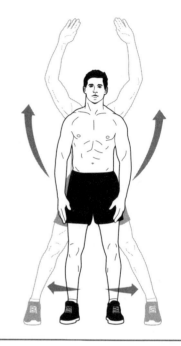

ARM CIRCLE
(10 IN EACH DIRECTION)
Stand upright and simultaneously swing both arms in large circles, allowing the shoulder blades to move freely. Perform 15 reps forward, then reverse the movement and perform 15 circling the arms backward.

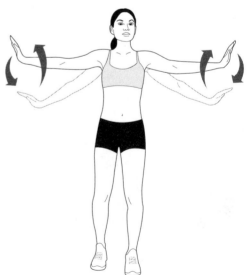

WALKING HIGH KNEES

Stand tall with your feet shoulder-width apart. Without changing your posture, raise your left knee as high as you can and step forward. Repeat with your right leg. Continue to alternate back and forth.

WALKING HIGH KICK

• Stand tall with your arms hanging at your sides. Keeping your knee straight, kick your left leg up—reaching with your right arm out to meet it— as you simultaneously take a step forward (just imagine that you're a Russian soldier).

• As soon as your left foot touches the floor, repeat the movement with your right leg and left arm. Alternate back and forth.

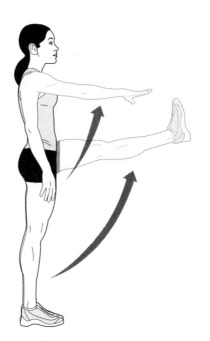

LUNGE WITH SIDE BEND

• Stand tall with your arms hanging at your sides. Step forward with your right leg and lower your body until your right knee is bent at least 90 degrees.

• As you lunge, reach over your head with your left arm as you bend your torso to your right. Reach for the floor with your right hand. Return to the starting position.

• Complete the prescribed number of reps, then lunge with your left leg and bend to your left for the same number of reps.

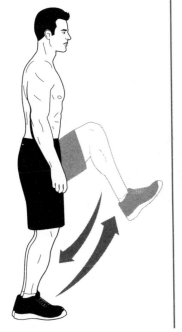

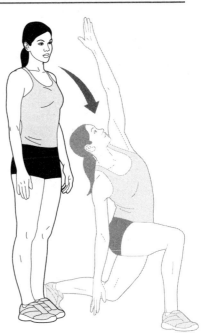

DYNAMIC STRETCHING AND WARMUP—*Continued*

REVERSE LUNGE WITH REACH BACK
(DUMBBELLS OPTIONAL)

• Stand tall with your arms hanging at your sides. Brace your core and hold it that way. Lunge back with your right leg, lowering your body until your left knee is bent at least 90 degrees.

• As you lunge, reach back over your shoulders and to the left. Reverse the movement back to the starting position.

• Complete the prescribed number of reps with your right leg, then step back with your left leg and reach over your right shoulder for the same number of reps. Keep your torso upright for the entire movement.

LOW SIDE-TO-SIDE LUNGE
(DUMBBELLS OPTIONAL)W

• Stand with your feet set about twice shoulder-length apart, your feet facing straight ahead. Clasp your hands in front of your chest (or hold dumbbells as shown).

• Shift your weight over to your right leg as you push your hips backward and lower your body by dropping your hips and bending your knees. Your lower right leg should remain nearly perpendicular to the floor. Your left foot should remain flat on the floor.

• Without raising yourself back up to a standing position, reverse the movement to the left. Alternate back and forth.

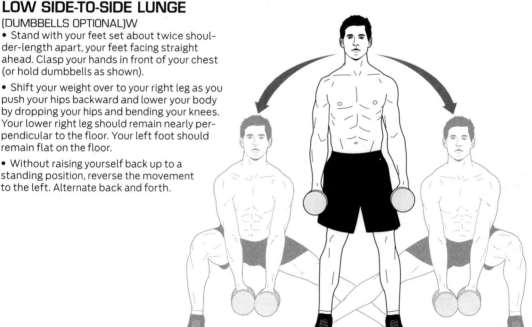

INVERTED HAMSTRING

• Stand on your right leg, your knee bent slightly. Raise your left foot slightly off the floor. Without changing the bend in your right knee, bend at your hips and lower your torso until it's parallel to the floor.

• As you bend over, raise your arms straight out from your sides until they're in line with your torso, your palms facing down. Your left leg should stay in line with your body as you lower your torso.

• Return to the start. Complete the prescribed number of repetitions on your right leg, then do the same number on your left.

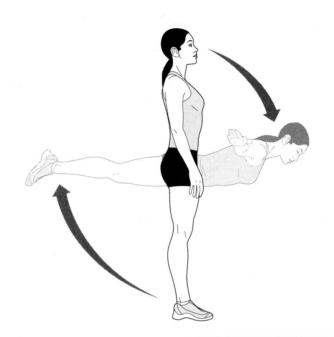

INCHWORM

• Stand tall with your legs straight and bend over and touch the floor. Keeping your legs straight, walk your hands forward (if you can't reach the floor with your legs straight, bend your knees just enough so you can. As your flexibility improves, try to straighten them a little more). Keeping your core braced, walk your hands out as far as you can without allowing your hips to sag.

• Then take tiny steps to walk your feet back to your hands. That's 1 repetition. Do 5 forward, and then 5 more in reverse.

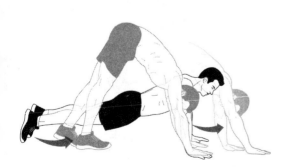

CARIOCA

(FAST, 25 STEPS IN EACH DIRECTION)
Assume an athletic stance—feet shoulder width apart and parallel, knees slightly bent—in an open field or aerobics room. Shift your weight onto the balls of your feet. Quickly cross your right foot in front of your left, then your left foot out to your left. On your next step, cross your right foot behind your left foot, then step your left foot to your left again. Continue moving to your left, alternating stepping your right foot in front of and behind your left. Repeat for 15 yards, then stop and reverse the movement, moving to your right in the same manner.

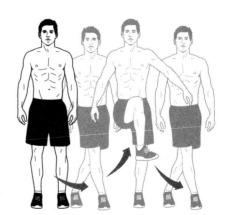

DYNAMIC STRETCHING AND WARMUP—*Continued*

DYNAMIC STRETCHING: ROUTINE #2

SINGLE-LEG GLUTE BRIDGE

Lie faceup on the floor with your left knee bent and your right leg straight. Raise your right leg until it's in line with your left thigh. Place your arms out to your sides at 45-degree angles to your torso, palms facing up. Push your hips upward, keeping your right leg elevated and in line with your left thigh. Be sure to push up from your heel (you can raise your toes to help). Your body should form a straight line from your shoulders to your knees. Pause, then slowly lower your body and leg back to the starting position. Halfway through the prescribed time, switch legs.

WALKING HIGH KICK

• Stand tall with your arms hanging at your sides. Keeping your knee straight, kick your left leg up—reaching with your right arm out to meet it—as you simultaneously take a step forward (just imagine that you're a Russian soldier).

• As soon as your left foot touches the floor, repeat the movement with your right leg and left arm. Alternate back and forth.

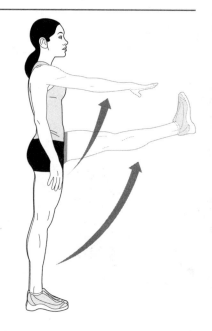

WALKING HIGH KNEES

Stand tall with your feet shoulder-width apart. Without changing your posture, raise your left knee as high as you can and step forward. Repeat with your right leg. Continue to alternate back and forth.

WALKING SPIDERMAN STRETCH (10 PER SIDE)

Assume a standard pushup position, hands under your shoulders, body straight, neck in line with the spine. Step your right foot forward and place it flat on the floor just outside your right hand (or as close to it as you can get comfortably). Pause for a 2-count, then walk your hands forward until you are back in the pushup position. Repeat the move, stepping your left foot forward, and repeat, moving down the floor, alternating sides for reps.

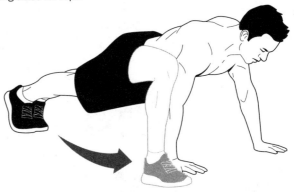

WALL SLIDE

Stand with your feet parallel and your heels, butt, upper back, and the back of your head touching a wall behind you. Extend your arms overhead so that the backs of your hands and elbows contact the wall behind you. Slowly bend your arms, sliding your elbows as far downward as you can while keeping the backs of your hands and elbows in contact with the wall. Reverse the movement, maintaining contact with the wall the whole time. That's 1 rep.

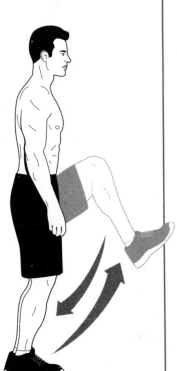

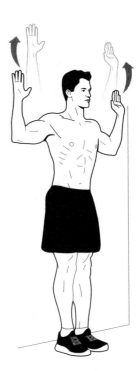

DYNAMIC STRETCHING AND WARMUP—*Continued*

STANDING Y, T, W, L, 5/STATION

Stand upright with your feet parallel and at shoulder width. Perform each of the following moves slowly five times each, contracting the back muscles strongly at the top of each move:

Y

Keeping your arms straight and your shoulders down, raise your arms as far as possible overhead, palms facing one another, so your body forms a "Y" shape. Pause in the top position, lower your arms, and repeat.

T

Without shrugging your shoulders, extend your arms directly out to your sides, parallel to the floor, palms down. Squeeze your shoulder blades down and back, then bring your palms together in front of you and repeat.

W

Keeping your arms straight, spread your fingers and rotate your palms outward until your thumbs point backward. Squeeze your shoulder blades down and together, pause, return to the starting position, and repeat.

L

Bend your elbows 90 degrees, palms facing upward. Keeping you elbows close to your sides, rotate your upper arms outward so your palms travel backward slightly. Squeeze your shoulder blades down and together, pause, return to the starting position, and repeat.

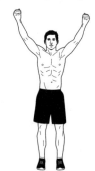 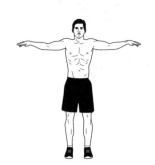 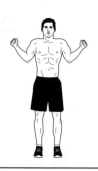 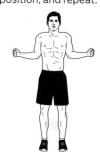

SQUAT THRUST

• Stand with your feet shoulder-width apart and your arms at your sides. Push your hips back, bend your knees, and lower your body as deep as you can into a squat.

• As you squat down, place your hands on the floor in front of you, shifting your weight onto them. Kick your legs backward, so that you're now in a pushup position.

• Quickly bring your legs back to the squat position. Stand up quickly and repeat the movement.

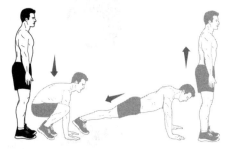

INCHWORM

• Stand tall with your legs straight and bend over and touch the floor. Keeping your legs straight, walk your hands forward (if you can't reach the floor with your legs straight, bend your knees just enough so you can. As your flexibility improves, try to straighten them a little more). Keeping your core braced, walk your hands out as far as you can without allowing your hips to sag.

• Then take tiny steps to walk your feet back to your hands. That's 1 repetition. Do 5 forward, and then 5 more in reverse.

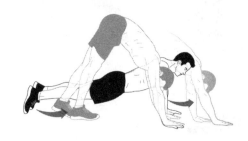

FORWARD-BACKWARD JUMP (20)

Assume a shoulder-width stance with your feet parallel. Keeping your gaze forward and your shoulders square, alternate jumping a few inches forward, then the same distance back, continuously for 30 reps.

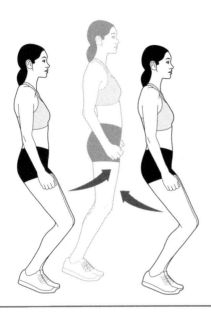

SIDE-TO-SIDE JUMP (20)

Assume a shoulder-width stance with your feet parallel. Keeping your gaze forward and your shoulders square, alternate jumping a few inches to your left, then the same distance to your right, continuously for 30 reps.

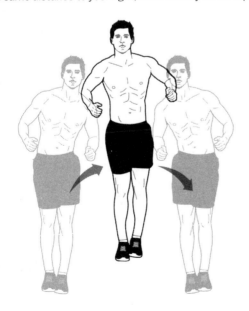

SPECIAL SECTION
The Posture Page

How can you make yourself feel more capable, more energetic, and healthier *instantly?* Improve your posture.

The body and the mind have a symbiotic relationship: Change one and you change the other. So in the long term, keeping your body healthy improves your outlook, and keeping a positive mental attitude helps keep your body healthy.

But this works in the short term as well: Researchers from Columbia University recently conducted an experiment in which they had subjects assume various postures that typically imply dominance: feet up, or leaning forward over a desk. The result? Not only did the subjects feel more powerful, their testosterone levels went up while their stress hormones went down—all in the space of about 15 minutes.

The converse is also true: When subjects slouched and crossed their arms, testosterone levels sank and stress levels rose.

The lesson here is not that you should strut like a peacock through your day—overcompensating probably won't have the same effect, and you'll probably look silly in the process. But our habitual posture clearly sends a strong message, not only to the people around us but to own our nervous system. And if you choose, you can take control over those neural signals, lifting your mood and brightening up your day a little at the same time. Health-wise, good posture makes a huge difference as well. Habitual chair-slouching plays hell on your neck, spine, and hip joints—and, eventually, on your internal organs as well.

How do you change your posture?

It's useful to remember that we all had perfect posture once, and that our skeletons are, in fact, built for walking, standing, and moving with perfect alignment. If you have young children, or nieces or nephews of your own, watch them sometime as they move through their day. Regardless of whether they're sitting, standing, squatting, walking, or running, their posture is close to perfect. It's not rigid, military posture: It's loose, graceful, and poised: dancer-like. You don't have to tell a 3-year-old to "sit up straight": Give them a firm, flat chair and something to do and they'll sit up straight effortlessly on their own.

Good posture in adults, then, shouldn't feel imposed. You don't achieve it by being tense. When you're moving well, paradoxically, the right posture can make you feel both more relaxed *and* more energized. You're giving your muscles a break and letting your skeleton do the work it's built for—to keep you aligned and upright with a minimum of conscious effort.

The workout programs in this book can help enormously in freeing you up from the habitual tension that causes bad posture. Walking and running, especially, help to tone the muscles you need to sit and stand straight, and, simultaneously, to lengthen and loosen tense areas that can pull you into a forward slouch.

Taking short work breaks every 20 to 25 minutes, changing your sitting position often, and staying physically active throughout your day—and not just during your workout—will also go a long way toward improving posture.

In addition, the following exercise, based on the work of engineer and somatic expert Dr. Moshe Feldenkrais, is specifically designed to free up the muscles around your hips, back, and shoulders and to ease the spine back into an optimal alignment. Take your time going through it, and perform the movement with as little effort as possible: The entire exercise should have a rag doll–like feel. Try it after waking up in the morning, before sleeping at night, or while taking a brief break from work: You'll feel more aligned, relaxed, and alert.

LYING SIDE WINDMILL

1. Lie on your back and close your eyes. Spend a moment settling into the floor and relaxing completely. Breathe normally.

2. Bend your legs so your feet can be flat on the floor, knees pointed toward the ceiling.

3. Allow your knees to fall to the left slightly, then to the right.

4. Repeat this movement several times, gradually increasing the range of motion so that your lower back twists gently.

5. Keeping your feet on the floor, allow your knees to fall as far as comfortably possible to your right. Don't stretch.

6. Extend your arms outward from your shoulders along the floor, palms up, so that they form right angles to your body.

7. Turn your head easily to your left, as if to look at your left hand.

8. With your left hand, slowly trace a large semicircle along the floor up over your head.
  Continue this movement until your left shoulder lifts from the floor, your left arm is lying on top of your right, and you are lying fully on your right side.

9. Keeping your knees to the right, slowly reverse that movement, tracing a half circle along the floor until your arms are once again fully extended 90 degrees out from your shoulders, palms up.

10. Repeat that movement eight times, then drop your knees to the left, your head to the right, and repeat for 8 reps on that side.

BRONZE
MONTH 3
CONGRATULATIONS, YOU MADE IT!

If you've been following the program up to now, you will have taken 60 walks of at least a half hour in length, done at least 15 foam-rolling sessions, and 15 dynamic-stretching and warmup sessions. Your muscles and connective tissue are far healthier than when you started. Everyday movement is probably easier and more fluid. You're almost certainly feeling better and looking better, and without a doubt you're healthier inside than when you started.

During your final month as a true beginner, you're going to kick things up another few notches. In fact, this is the level at which you transition from being a casual exerciser to the person who's in it for lasting, visible, long-term results.

As you'll see, this section contains a lot more information than previous months: more specific directives, more exercises. At the same time, you'll also have more choice about how you spend your exercise time—solace for those of you who were getting tired of walking!—and even, at the end of the chapter, an option to start getting into organized competition. That's a little further incentive to be extra focused during this crucial 4-week period in the program.

There are going to be three major additions to the program this month:

1. Two strength-training sessions per week

2. More intense cardio work and

3. As much additional activity as you can get into your day, in the form of active rest and NEAT.

This month, with some variation, your workout weeks are going to look like this:

YOUR BRONZE MONTH 3 ROUTINE

MONDAY:	Foam rolling, dynamic warmup, strength-training workout #1
TUESDAY:	20 minutes moderate-intensity cardio activity of choice
WEDNESDAY:	40-minute walk or low-intensity cardio of choice
THURSDAY:	Foam rolling, dynamic warmup, strength-training workout #2
FRIDAY:	Dynamic warmup, 20 minutes moderate-intensity cardio
SATURDAY:	40-minute walk *or* low-intensity cardio *or* 20-minute moderate-intensity cardio
SUNDAY:	Foam rolling, 40-minute walk *or* low-intensity cardio *or* 20 minutes moderate-intensity cardio *or* active rest and NEAT

Sound like a lot? Don't sweat the sweat: Despite these additions, your time commitment this month will be roughly the same as it was last month—no more than about 30 or 40 minutes a day.

Strength Training

A hundred (or so) years ago, strength training was largely the domain of professional strongmen who paraded around vaudeville stages in lion skins. Just a few short decades ago, coaches warned athletes to stay away from strength training lest it bind them up and slow them down. No longer: The benefits of resistance training are so well accepted now that most medical professionals recommend that all their patients do some form of it at least twice a week. The American College of Sports Medicine makes a similar recommendation.

Why the change? The 1968 publication of Dr. Kenneth Cooper's book, *Aerobics,* spurred a slew of research on endurance-type exercise. And the results, naturally enough, were encouraging: Virtually everyone who exercised in that manner got healthier. But at the same time, more strenuous forms of exercise, like strength training, were largely ignored by the medical community. Part of this was practical. It's fairly easy, after all, to put someone on an exercise bike or a treadmill, hook them up to various monitors, and track how they

respond. It's comparatively tougher to track someone's vital signs while they traipse around the weight room.

Starting 20 years ago, however, additional research began pouring in about how strength training could provide different benefits that may be equally—if not more—important than those derived from aerobic training. As it turned out, strength work afforded exercisers many of the same benefits that came from cardio work: heart and lungs got stronger, blood pressure dropped, glucose metabolism improved. At the same time, strength training elicited additional changes *not* typically associated with aerobic exercise: more muscle mass; more strength and mobility; denser, stronger bones; better body composition.

Muscle mass is the engine of youth: Sedentary adults typically lose it at a rate of about 1 percent per year after the age of 40. The resulting loss of strength eventually reduces mobility and increases the chances of falling and injury during day-to-day activities. It's harder to get in and out of a chair, tougher to turn your head to see behind you in the car. Immobility then creates a vicious cycle: The less you move, the less you *want* to move, and the faster you lose your mobility—and your muscle. With less muscle tissue around to burn through calories, the chances of obesity and diabetes also shoot up as well.

As beneficial as it is, low-intensity aerobic exercise doesn't protect you against this age-related decline in

THE MYSTERY OF THE NONRESPONDER

Between the lines of just about every well-documented study on the effects of exercise is a dirty little secret: Although the vast majority of people benefit from resistance and aerobic exercise—improving health markers, building muscle, and so on—some unfortunate people don't respond at all.

Jamie Timmons, a professor of systems biology at the Royal Veterinary College in London, estimates that as much as 20 percent of the population may be "nonresponders" to standard exercise.

What's behind this mystery? Unsurprisingly, genetics play a role: Timmons and his colleagues found 29 genes that appeared to be linked to exercise nonresponsiveness. Diet, stress, and living environment may play an as-yet-undetermined role as well. But Timmons's major conclusion for the average fitness enthusiast is that, when it comes to exercise, one size doesn't necessarily fit all.

As I've written elsewhere in this book, the body always responds very specifically to exercise, rising to meet the exact demands you place on it. It's possible, then, that nonresponders may not be nonresponders at all—just unresponsive to the specific types of exercise they've already tried.

With more experimentation, they may well find some form of exercise that works better for them.

So if you haven't responded well to exercise in the past, you may do well to continue hunting around for an approach that you enjoy—and from which you can derive maximal benefit. I wholly stand by the effectiveness of the workouts in this book, and they will be effective for the vast majority of people who undertake them. But I'll also be the first to admit that even the workouts I recommend won't necessarily clinch it for absolutely everyone: How you respond to them, as to any workout program, is going to be a product of your genetics, your diet, your environment, and how hard you work at it.

But even if you never find the magic formula that builds you the sleek musculature and the tour-de-France-worthy cardiovascular system you've always dreamed about, never give up on exercise. Regardless of your genetics, if you're working out regularly, you're still almost certainly deriving many (if not all) of the dozens of physiological, psychological, and physical benefits available through regular exercise—and, quite possibly, even a few we haven't yet learned how to measure.

strength. The body always responds *specifically* to exercise—it gets better at whatever you ask of it, but not at what you don't. So a slow, long-distance exerciser like a jogger gets better at moving slowly over long distances, but not better at lifting heavy objects or moving quickly.

Regular strength trainers, however, do get stronger and faster, and they do gain muscle mass and mobility at the same time.

Perhaps most significantly, though, strength training causes self-esteem, body image, and confidence to soar—and the value of those changes can't be overstated. As a doctor, I'm of course very concerned about health markers like blood pressure numbers and glucose metabolism—factors that profoundly affect longevity and long-term quality of life. But at the same time, I understand that unless you've got heart disease or diabetes, those numbers don't mean anywhere near as much to you as how you feel about yourself walking around in your own skin, 24-7. You can't put a cocktail dress or a tailored suit on a 110/60 blood pressure reading or a stellar blood-lipid profile.

Unless you work at it for a long time, the visible changes you get from aerobic training are fairly subtle: You're a little leaner, a little more toned. But most people who begin regular strength training—and work hard at it—see some pretty substantial improvements in how they look after just a few weeks. And if you're diligent about it, those improvements can keep coming to the point that pretty soon you'll want a new wardrobe to show off all your hard work.

You're not going to turn into Superman or Venus Williams with a few weeks of training. But you *will* become a leaner and more athletic version of you—and it may well happen sooner than you think.

Your choices for strength training extend far beyond old-school barbells and dumbbells—though these standbys are still great choices. Bodyweight training, kettlebells, gymnastics-style training, Olympic-style lifting, and suspension training all fulfill the strength-training portion of the workout.

This month, however, you're going to use only your body weight for strength training: No need for any equipment—or even a gym.

How Fit Am I? A 6-Minute Self-Test

Before you embark on your third—and final—month of this program, I want you to take an informal reading of your current fitness level. I have no doubt you'll feel far better 4 weeks from now, subjectively speaking, than you do now. This test, however, will give you objective proof that you're stronger, faster, and fitter than when you started.

After a brief dynamic stretching warmup, do as many full reps as you can with good form in the time indicated. *Be honest and don't count partial reps.* Go strictly by the clock. Take 3 minutes' complete rest between exercises.

- **MAXIMUM BODY-WEIGHT SQUATS** in 40 seconds: Descend until the tops of your thighs are parallel with the floor.

- **MAXIMUM PUSHUPS** in 40 seconds: hands elevated or on the floor, depending on your level of fitness. On the floor: Descend to 4 inches—or one fist's width—from the floor. Elevated: Touch chest to the platform.

- **MAXIMUM PRONE SWIMS** in 40 seconds: Lie on your stomach with your arms extended overhead and your back arched so your head is off the floor. Keeping your arms straight and your hands off the floor, bring your hands toward your sides as if performing a prone jumping-jack. Return to the starting position. That's 1 rep.

Make a note of the number of reps you do on each move. Towel off and go take your walk for the day.

MONTH 3
BODY-WEIGHT WORKOUTS

Now that you have a benchmark down, it's time to get going on improving on it. Choose 2 nonconsecutive days during the week—say, Monday and Thursday—and do one of the following workouts on each of those 2 days.

On the days when you strength train, start with the foam-rolling routine, move on to one of the two dynamic-warmup routines from last month (your choice), and then hit up one of the two following strength-training sessions.

All three parts of the workout should take you 40 minutes or less. On each workout, perform the exercises for a total of 40 seconds. Rest for 20 seconds, then move on to the next exercise. Take a 1-minute break, then perform the entire cycle two more times, for a total work time of about 20 minutes.

Work as hard as you can during those 40-second intervals, doing as many reps as possible. If your form starts to break down, pause for a moment—but keep the clock running. As you get stronger, you'll be able to keep working at a steady pace throughout the entire 40-second time period.

WORKOUT #1

PLANK
Get into pushup position, but bend your elbows and rest your weight on your forearms. Your body should form a straight line from your shoulders to your ankles. Brace your core and hold.

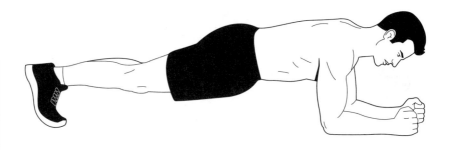

SQUAT
Place your fingers on the back of your head and pull your elbows back so that they're in line with your body. Squat until your thighs are parallel to the floor, pause for a second, then push back to the starting position.

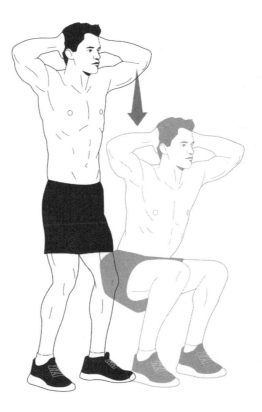

WALKING LUNGE

Perform a lunge, but instead of pushing your body
backward to the starting position, rise up and bring
your back foot forward so that you move forward
(like you're walking) a step with every rep. Alternate
the leg you step forward with each time.

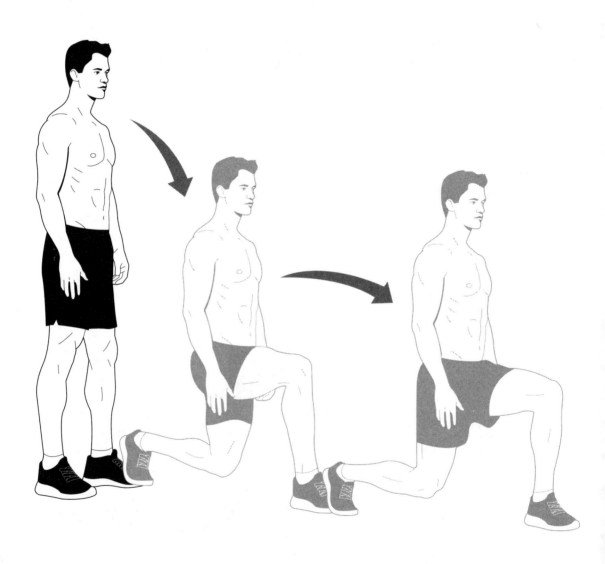

COBRA

• Lie facedown on the floor with your legs straight and your arms next to your sides, palms down.

• Contract your glutes and the muscles of your lower back and raise your head, chest, arms, and legs off the floor.

• Simultaneously rotate your arms so that your thumbs point toward the ceiling. At this time, your hips should be the only parts of your body touching the floor. Hold this position for the prescribed time.

NOTE: If you can't hold it for the entire time, hold for 5 to 10 seconds, rest for 5, and repeat as many times as needed. If the exercise is too easy, you can hold light dumbbells in your hands while you do it.

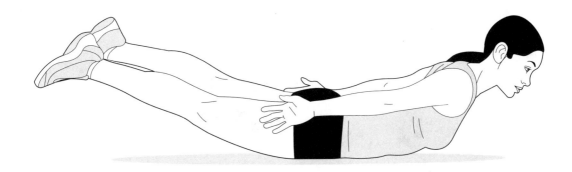

PUSHUP

Get into pushup position using your hands as a base, if you want to make it more interesting. Keeping your body straight from your head to your ankles, lower your body until your chest nearly touches the floor. Pause at the bottom and then push yourself back to the starting position as quickly as possible.

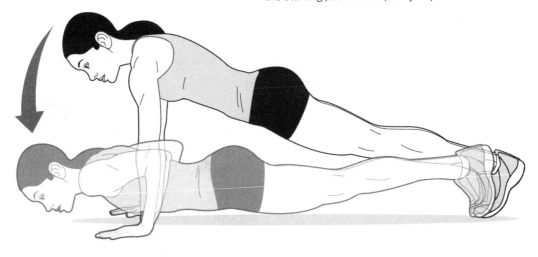

WORKOUT #2

SIDE PLANK
Lie on your side and use your forearm to support your body. Raise your hips until your body forms a straight line from shoulder to ankles. Hold and repeat for other side.

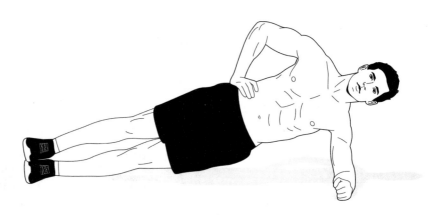

LUNGE WITH REAR FOOT ELEVATED
(Perform 40 seconds on each side with a 20-second rest between.)

• Place a pad on the floor, about 1 foot in front of a knee-high bench or aerobic step. Stand with your back 2 to 3 feet from the step. Extend your left leg behind you, positioning your knee above the pad, and rest as much of the top of your foot as is comfortable on the step.

• Keeping your torso upright, bend both legs, slowly dropping your left knee toward the floor and stopping when your knee lightly touches the pad. Pushing down through the heel of your right foot, return to the starting position and repeat for reps.

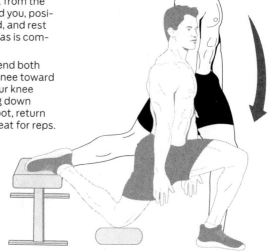

PUSH-BACK PUSHUP

From the pushup position, lower your chest toward the floor, keeping your body straight, head to heels. As you push yourself back up, allow you knees to bend and your butt to travel toward the ceiling as you push the floor forward and away from you (it should feel as if you are performing an overhead press). At the top of the move, your knees should be bent and your body should form a straight line from your hands to your tailbone. Slowly return to the bottom of the pushup position and repeat for reps.

ALTERNATING SINGLE-LEG GLUTE BRIDGE

Lie faceup on the floor with your left knee bent and your right leg straight. Raise your right leg until it's in line with your left thigh. Place your arms out to your sides at 45-degree angles to your torso, palms facing up. Push your hips upward, keeping your right leg elevated and in line with your left thigh. Be sure to push up from your heel (you can raise your toes to help). Your body should form a straight line from your shoulders to your knees. Pause, then slowly lower your body and leg back to the starting position. Alternate legs after each rep.

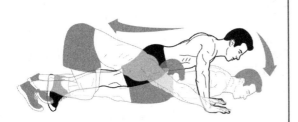
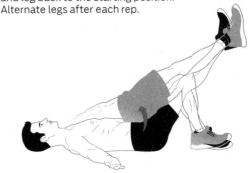

PRONE SWIM

Lie on your stomach with your arms extended overhead and your back arched so your head is off the floor. Keeping your arms straight and your hands off the floor, bring your hands toward your sides as if performing a prone jumping-jack. Return to the starting position. That's 1 rep.

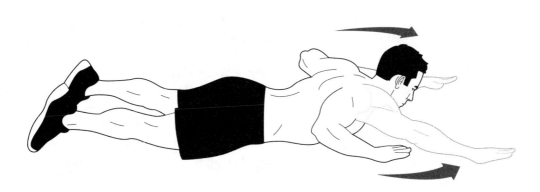

MONTH 3
EXPANDING YOUR CARDIO HORIZONS

The term "cardio" or "aerobic exercise" covers a pretty broad swath of different activities. Essentially it's any physical activity you can do continuously, for 20 minutes or more, that drives your heart rate up to at least 60 percent of your maximal heart rate. (You can find that number—*very roughly*—by subtracting your age from 220. But for simplicity's sake, you can also use the chart I gave you in the last chapter.) As I'll discuss later, continuous, low-intensity exercise isn't the *only* way to exercise your cardiovascular system, but it's a tried and true way, it's very safe and effective, and so for now, it's the method I suggest you use.

Up to this point in the program, you've been walking every day for cardio exercise. Some people will want to stop there—and that's fine, as long as you keep your intensity up at the recommended levels. Thousands of people have lost tons of weight doing it.

This month, however, I'm going to expand your horizons a bit: Now that you've established a regular rhythm for working out in your life, I want to let you choose *how* to exercise your heart and lungs.

What type of cardio is best for you? I'm going to remind you of commandment one: *Thou Shalt Have Fun.* Choose something you love! Choosing your cardio is a little like choosing a major in college: Where do your interests lie? What are you good at? What can you spend lots of time doing without getting bored or distracted? This may be the most important step in your quest for fitness, so take it seriously.

If you don't know yet, that's okay. Give something a try, and if you hate it, change it up till you find something you like more. If that becomes boring 3 months later, change it up again. And again. Then cycle back to the thing you did first. As I'll explain in a moment, there's a lot of value in variety.

But for now, you need a place to start, an activity to focus on. There are a lot of choices out there, from outdoor group sports like soccer to solitary indoor pursuits like using the elliptical machine. All have pluses and minuses. Here's a rundown of some of the most popular:

WALKING

Pros: Some fitness folks say we were born to run. I agree! I love it. But I also I say we were born to walk. Walking is the number-one choice for beginners, and can continue to be a standby for your whole exercise career. Anyone with two legs (and some with fewer) can do it; it's calming, invigorating, balancing. It clears your mind and gives you focus like no other type of exercise. Added to that, it's convenient—you can walk virtually anywhere, anytime. As mentioned above, most people who get lots of NEAT do so through walking.

It's effective exercise as well: The National Weight Control Registry lists walking as the number one physical activity used by people who successfully lose substantial amounts of weight—and keep it off.

Cons: The only downside to walking is that, very quickly, it ceases to be truly aerobic: Our skeletons, rather than our muscles, do much of the work while we walk, and so many people can walk for long periods without breaking a sweat, much less getting their heart rate into the aerobic zone. Walk regularly for a few weeks and this is likely to become the case for you too.

When that happens, you can pick up the pace or start walking on more challenging terrain (you may have already started to do that). Now that you're in month 3, you could also carry something heavy while you walk: a pair of dumbbells, a loaded backpack, or, if you've got one handy, a child in a carrier (who says you can't exercise when you have kids?). One very athletic guy I know sometimes walks around his block carrying 50-pound kettlebells—an advanced and challenging workout, even for someone who's already in great shape.

The Verdict: More walking is almost always a good idea, and if you like, it can become your primary mode of aerobic exercise, now and forever. I can't recommend it enough—or enough *of* it.

RUNNING

Pros: I run. A lot. I dream about running, and sometimes feel like I'm dreaming while I'm running. I compete as a runner, and it's also one major tool I use to keep in shape.

What's so great about running? It burns a lot of calories, for one thing: a 180-pound man can burn 700 calories an hour running at 6 miles an hour on the flat—that's a lot. Running is convenient and fun—there's almost nothing I like better than getting acquainted with a city I'm visiting by taking a run through its streets. And on a basic level, it's a primitive movement that doesn't require coaching, equipment, or specialized training: You just lace up your shoes and go. Running is always there for you, always a possibility. That's why I love it. And yet . . .

Cons: I'm going to qualify my recommendation of running for the average, or beginning, exerciser. Primarily, it's because running is tough on your joints. Every time your foot lands, the muscles and bones of the landing foot have to absorb a force equal to at least four times your body weight. No matter how sylphlike your form, or delicate your physique, this is a tremendous pressure for your feet, knees, ankles, hips, and back to endure, and it causes a lot of injuries over time: A 2007 study determined that at least one in five runners get injured at some point throughout their running careers.

Too often, rank beginners go out on day one, try to run 2 miles, wake up in agony the next day, and swear off exercise forever. Or, worse, they think they're up for running a marathon with just a few weeks of training (I strongly discourage this approach!).

Don't add your name to the casualty list by going from zero to miles of running at a time in your first week, especially if you're new to exercise or overweight. Walk first, then alternate periods of walking with short periods of slow running, and gradually build it up (add up your total running mileage for the week and don't exceed that number by more than 10 percent the following week). The impact that running generates can be a good thing, causing your bones to become denser and more resilient. Just use any unusual soreness, pain, or discomfort as a sign that you did too much, and back off.

Your body *will* adapt to long-distance running. You just need to give yourself time to build up. As the saying goes, don't run to get in shape. Get in shape, then run.

A good pair of shoes is invaluable for running as well. If you're serious about running, take the time to get properly fitted at a running-specific store, and make the investment in a good pair.

The Verdict: Great to do once you're in shape to handle it. Beginners, use caution.

SWIMMING

Pros: Swimming and other water-based activities like pool aerobic classes are a terrific option for people with arthritis and other movement limitations: A 2011 study found that adults with hip and knee arthritis received similar boosts in mobility, function, and other health outcomes as they did from land-based rehabilitation. Swimming is low-impact, so stress fractures from swimming, common for runners, are virtually unheard-of. And swimming rarely makes you sore.

Swimming is also a skill that you can develop and refine; beginners who take a few lessons from a qualified coach often improve their endurance, speed, and efficiency very quickly. To me, it's nice to know that if I found myself stuck in the water a mile or more from shore, I could probably make my way back to land under my own power. Though many people just go to a pool and do lap after lap, I've always enjoyed the interval-style pool training preferred by many coaches, which can build strength and muscle as well as endurance, particularly in the upper body.

Cons: Chlorine hair, anyone? Pool swimming can definitely be hard on your skin, eyes, and hair. It's also not the most convenient activity: You need a pool or, failing that, a lake, river, or pond with an attentive lifeguard, decent weather, and a place to shower and change afterward. And there are, of course, dangers associated with swimming—especially in the ocean—that you need to be aware of, and the possibility of swimmer's ear, and impingement or overuse injuries in the shoulders.

The Verdict: As long as it's convenient for you, go for it—just learn how to do it right first.

CYCLING

Pros: Speed, exhilaration, being at one with nature and a well-tuned machine, zipping past commuters stuck in traffic and turning *your* commute into a pulse-pounding, low-impact adventure—what's not to love about cycling?

Cons: Well . . . a couple of things: It's a gear-heavy pursuit, for one thing. If you're serious about it, be prepared to drop close to a grand on everything you need, including shoes, helmet, duds, and the bike itself, and to spend a few bucks a year (or some time, if you're so inclined) keeping everything tuned up. It can be dangerous, and you need a place to do it: Fighting traffic is okay if you're up for it, but there's really

nothing like the open road for a good cycling workout.

Cycling can also eat up a fair amount of time: A beginner in reasonable shape can work up to cycling for 90 minutes or more pretty quickly. Add that to the likely necessity of driving to and from your start point, and you're looking at a 2-hour time commitment, minimum, for a decent ride. For that reason, most cyclists save their serious riding for the weekends.

Finally, though it's great for your entire body—especially your legs—cycling can be rough on your posture, and potentially, rougher on your bones. The seated, forward-leaning posture that cycling requires is not too far afield from the infamous desk-sitting position that we should all be trying to do less of. And a 2009 study indicated that competitive cycling may *lower* bone density—leaving you more at risk for bone fractures.

The Verdict: If you've got the time for it, and crave a little speed, there's nothing like it. Just make sure to supplement your training with plenty of stretching and weight-bearing activities so your bones get a workout too.

INDOOR CARDIO MACHINES

Pros: I'm lumping these into one category because their pros and cons are all virtually identical: On the pro side, they're convenient and, for the most part, safe. Fixed-foot units like the elliptical trainer, the StairMaster, the Arc Trainer, the TreadClimber, and the VersaClimber are low-impact, so you don't need to worry about running-type injuries. You can see how far you've gone, how many calories you've burned, and the METs (metabolic equivalents) you've achieved (though those numbers can be unreliable). If it's cold out, or if being outside is otherwise inconvenient, these machines can be a huge benefit.

Cons: You're stuck indoors, for starters, and that's a disadvantage right there. A 2008 study found that outdoor exercise in a natural setting had a 50 percent greater positive effect on mental health than working out at the gym. Additionally, there's a good chance you'll wind up staring at a digital readout of your progress or, worse, at a TV screen while at the gym—and screen time is another thing we probably don't need more of. On fixed-foot machines, the movement of your limbs is dictated by the machines, rather than your own ergonomics, and that can potentially be rough on your joints over time.

As you can see, I'm not a huge fan. But convenience is a huge plus, particularly during winter months. If you like indoor cardio workouts, or the weather is making an outdoor workout impossible, choose a free-foot machine, like a treadmill or StepMill (which resembles a downward-moving escalator). These machines give you a better workout,

and their movements more closely mimic the functional, true-life movements of running and climbing stairs.

The Verdict: An acceptable, safe, and low-impact option if you can't make it outside.

GROUP CLASSES: ZUMBA, STEP, BOOT CAMPS, MARTIAL ARTS, CROSSFIT

Pros: If you're into a group dynamic, these classes are fantastic. Some people get very attached to their instructors and fellow classmates and develop a whole social routine surrounding the class, which can be very motivating and supportive (as long as it doesn't involve stopping for a chocolate scone and a venti Frappuccino afterward). Good instructors keep things fresh and exciting, and can help you monitor any injuries and limitations that come up. If you're learning a skill—such as in a dance or martial arts class—they'll keep you learning, advancing, and exercising your brain as well, which is an undervalued aspect of exercise.

If you've never tried a group class, you may be surprised how hard they can be and how much harder you work with 50 other people in the room motivating you! Studies also indicate that listening to music (a frequent practice in these classes) while exercising at a moderate intensity can amp up both your intensity and enjoyment of exercise.

Cons: There is a big variation in quality of instruction in these classes, from one to the next. Some instructors are very knowledgeable (drop in on my weekend class sometime and you'll have an MD for an instructor!), others much less so. Depending on the focus and skill level of the students in the class, you may find yourself underchallenged or, equally, overwhelmed. Some instructors, notably those at Cross-Fit and some boot-camp-themed classes, pride themselves on being "hardcore" at all costs—which can be great for some people, terrible for others.

Fortunately, most classes grow by word of mouth, so you'll probably have a good sense of what you're getting into before you walk through the door. And terrible classes with incompetent instructors don't tend to last very long.

The Verdict: Check out the class or ask around. Once you know it's what you want, jump in.

SPORTS

Pros: Before there were stationary bikes and Spin classes, there were sports, and for some people, it starts and ends there. I know people who couldn't motivate themselves to step on a treadmill to save their lives; put a ball in front of them, however, and they're charging around for hours like a kid on a playground.

If you're in decent shape and haven't touched sports since middle school, I'd strongly advise getting into one if you can, even if you play just a few times a year. They're a great way to combine exercise and social bonding, to get to know new people or improve a group dynamic with people you already know or work with.

As with group classes, there's a large array of choices out there, from softball clubs to Ultimate Frisbee to soccer and rugby. Some individual sports—like tennis, racquetball, marathon, and triathlon—can morph into group activities if you do them with a club or league. I enjoy long runs and rides by myself, but I get a huge boost from working out alongside equally fierce competitors—to say nothing of racing against them!

Cons: Not all sports are truly aerobic in nature, or can even be considered exercise. Play an hour of full-court pickup basketball and you will probably cover 4 miles on foot, not to mention countless jumps and grabs and lunges and passes. Lawn bowling? Not so much.

Some sports carry risk of injury, of course. You're dealing with lots of random moving bodies scrambling for an elusive spherical object, so the sports environment is naturally more chaotic than a controlled gym workout. I see lots of torn ACLs and

BRONZE-LEVEL TRAINING: WHEN TO CALL A DOCTOR

There's a very good chance you'll get a little sore this month, with the new strength-training routine and intensified cardio. Sore is okay. It's normal. You definitely shouldn't feel yourself getting slower, weaker, or less energetic. If you do, and you're not sick or sleep-deprived, take a day or two off—and you'll probably be fine.

The red flag to watch out for in your workouts is *poor mechanics:* If your walking or running gait has changed—particularly if that change is asymmetrical, as in limping—you should go see a doctor, as you may have an orthopedic issue that needs attention.

sprained ankles from basketball, for example. Use your best judgment as to what sports you should participate in, at what level, and how often, and you should avoid any major trouble.

Those points aside, the inconvenience of figuring out where to meet and who will be there and who will bring the bat and ball is about the only downside of sports.

The Verdict: Keep an open-door policy to sports throughout your life based on what's available and interesting to you at any given time.

This is by no means a comprehensive list: Depending on where you are and the time of year, you can also

BRONZE-LEVEL BONUS: GOING FOR IT IN COMPETITION

At this point, some people finishing up the Bronze Level—maybe former athletes gradually gaining ground on their old level of fitness—will be itching for a way to show off their new strength and endurance in competition of some kind. If you participate in club sports, you may be doing that already.

For other people, who may be less enthusiastic about going public with their new fitness habit, I'm going to make a plug here that you do it now. Not necessarily for the competition itself, but to have a goal—something concrete that you're moving toward.

I understand being hesitant: By the time this book hits the shelf, I will have done 10 Ironman competitions—and those races still scare me a little. Over the 140 miles of an Ironman, nearly anything can happen: dehydration, pulled muscles, heat exhaustion, flat tires. The nervousness I feel about tackling that race is just enough to get me out on my bike for hours at a time on the week-

ends, just enough to get me out on the road for miles and miles, and just enough to get me swimming those endless laps in the pool on weekday mornings. Sure, I'd work out anyway (as I've said, I'm that kind of guy), but it wouldn't *matter* as much. Having the race in front of me keeps me on my toes—which in turn keeps me motivated and enthused.

So here's your final—optional— mission this month: Sign up for a 5-K. That's just over 3 miles, and if you've been keeping track, it's probably right around the amount you've been covering in your running workouts (if you've chosen to run) or your longer walks. In other words—it probably isn't as big a deal as you think.

Get yourself some good shoes (an essential investment), hit up some friends, and walk or walk-jog those 3 miles at an easy pace. Get a free T-shirt. Raise some money for a worthy cause. And celebrate your new fitness.

hike, climb mountains, cross-country
ski, mountain bike, kayak, stand-up
paddleboard, windsurf, and participate in any number of very enjoyable
activities. I'm of the general opi...
that if you're outside...
your heart rate is u...
probably a thumbs-u...
much the better!

of your thighs are parallel with the
floor.

• **Maximum Pushups** in 40 sec-
...nds: hands elevated or on the
...or, depending on your level of
...ess. On the floor: Descend to
...ches—or one fist's width—from
...loor. Elevated: Touch chest to
...atform.

Final Bron...
Level Gut C...

...imum **Prone Swims** in
...nds: Lie on your stomach
...r arms extended overhead
...back arched so your head
...loor. Keeping your arms
...d your hands off the
...your hands toward your
...erforming a prone
...Return to the starting
...'s 1 rep.

If you've completed all 12 w...
the Bronze-Level workout, i...
to take your temperature onc...
Pull out your scores from earl...
this month and repeat the sam...
exactly the same way. Here it is

After a brief dynamic stretc...
warmup, do as many full reps as...
can with good form in the time i...
cated. *Be honest and don't count pa...
reps.* Go strictly by the clock. Take...
3 minutes' complete rest between...
exercises.

...a note of your score:
...e going to be pleas-
...ess test periodi-
...is program—and
...n your computer
...dates on these
...ile will become
...y along the

• **Maximum Body-weight Squats** in
40 seconds: Descend until the tops

SILVER

THE INTERMEDIATE PROGRAM:
MONTHS 4–6

Many exercisers will start at this level. Maybe you're a former high school jock who's lost a few steps; maybe you never quite made it fully to jock status but tried on occasion. Maybe you're a fair-weather exerciser who's never quite gotten into a full-blown program. If that's the case with you, prepare to be pleasantly surprised: The boost of the occasional workout is nothing compared to the slow-but-steady improvements in health, fitness, and appearance that occur from months on a well-thought-out workout plan. These improvements start to feel like "the new normal" rather than some anomaly. You move, feel, and look different. I see that kind of shift all the time in people from all walks of life, and the transformation is impressive.

Meanwhile, if you're coming to the Silver Level from Bronze, you have an advantage, because you've already put in 80 to 90 workouts. You're already used to setting the time aside, and your habit is fully established. It's hard to overstate the importance of that. In the last section I recommended putting your workout in your day planner. If you've found that helpful up to now, continue. If you're new to the program, start now: Your workout is the most important appointment of the day.

Introducing Hybrid Workouts

What are you working today? Once you've been around the workout block a few times, this question comes up more and more.

Like many workout programs, the Bronze schedule is broken up into "strength-training" and "cardio" sessions: Some days you do one, some days you do another. Ask the average gym goer about their workouts and they'll probably describe something similar: "On Mondays, Wednesdays, and Fridays I'll do weights, and on Tuesdays and Thursdays I run on a treadmill." This fragmented approach is reflected in the layout of most commercial gyms as well: Cardio equipment is all in one area, weights are in another, and any large, open space, where one might run or sprint or carry or push something heavy, is somewhere else entirely. Gyms seem to reflect and encourage isolating parts and functions of the body:

"You're here to build bulky muscles or you're here to run a marathon," they seem to say. "If you want to do both or combine them, or do something in between, well . . . we don't know what to do with you."

I'm all for people exercising in whatever way they see fit—and any exercise program that gets you fired up and working out regularly is a huge positive. But I believe that trying to work the cardiovascular system in isolation from the muscles isn't all that practical or realistic. After all, the heart beats fast and you breathe fast during exercise *because* your muscles are working hard. Similarly, without the cardiovascular system to fuel them with oxygen and nutrients, your muscles wouldn't work at all.

Equally, I don't think programs that divvy up the body like dotted lines on a butcher's diagram—arms one day, chest the next, and so on—are a very good use of your time. These programs require you to do a high volume of exercise for one part

WANT BETTER, STRONGER WORKOUTS? READ THIS.

Starting the Silver Level is also a good time, if you haven't already, to flip to Part 4 and look at the eating tips for this program. As you become more active, you'll start to notice the relationship between what you eat and how you feel and perform in your workouts. That's a very good thing and a first step in getting you to shift your perspective on food from "something that fills me" to "something that fuels me."

of the body in a single day and are designed solely to bulk up the muscles. This is great if you're a bodybuilder, but that's a very specific training goal, and not what we're going after here.

Also, if you're trying to beat your personal record in a marathon, or clean-and-jerk the most weight at your gym's Olympic weightlifting competition, you're going to need to train specifically for that event. Endurance runners need to focus on running, weightlifters on lifting. There are entire books and coaching programs dedicated to training programs for just this sort of event.

One cool thing about the body—which you'll discover the longer you work out—is that it can adapt to virtually anything you throw at it. Start lifting weights seriously and you'll pack on muscles and get stronger. Start running a lot, and your heart and lungs will get more efficient to make you better at that. As you try different sports and activities throughout your athletic career, you can experiment and watch the different ways in which your body adapts to the different stimuli.

But unless you've already fallen in love with a particular sport, you probably aren't after any specific kind of fitness, but rather a blend of strength and endurance, and a blend of athletic muscularity and leanness. You want to be able to go on a long hike one day, play a rousing game of tag with your nieces and nephews the next, and help move a couch the day after. And you don't want to wake up the next morning feeling like you've been hit by a brick wall. In other words, you want *functional* strength and fitness: fitness that's applicable to an almost infinite number of sport and real-life situations.

Not only does functional fitness promote glowing health, head to toe and inside and out, it's also the perfect foundation that you need to build should you ever decide to specialize in a particular sport, be it running, weight lifting, tennis, dance, or the martial arts. A solid base of general fitness will put you at a huge advantage on virtually any playing field.

To that end, now that you're at the Silver Level, you're going to take more of a "hybrid" approach to nearly all your workouts. Strength-training workouts will now affect your heart and lungs, and feel a little more like cardio workouts; many of the cardio workouts will tax your muscles in ways that will probably feel more like training for strength. Every workout, to a certain degree, will help you build muscle, improve your cardiovascular system, *and* help you burn fat.

That's one-stop shopping and incredibly time-efficient. And when someone at the gym asks you, "What are you working today?" you can just say, "Everything!"

MONTH 1

During each week of the first month of Silver-Level training, you'll do two hybrid strength-training sessions, one or two interval sessions, one or two moderate-intensity cardio sessions, and two easy walks. Continue to foam-roll three times a week, and perform one of the dynamic warmup sequences, described in the previous chapter, before all workouts (they aren't necessary before your walks).

Do seven workouts a week, and never do the same type of workout 2 days in a row. The one exception to this last rule is the easy walk (or bike ride, or hike), which I encourage you to take not only when it's scheduled but whenever you have the time and energy—even if it's just 10 minutes at a time. Continue to do as much NEAT—*nonexercise activity thermogenesis*—such as housework, gardening, playing with kids, as you can. See the previous chapter for tips on this.

So a week of workouts might look like this:

YOUR SILVER MONTH 1 ROUTINE

MONDAY:	Strength training
TUESDAY:	Interval training
WEDNESDAY:	Easy walk
THURSDAY:	Strength training
FRIDAY:	Moderate cardio
SATURDAY:	Interval training
SUNDAY:	Easy walk

If you'd prefer to avoid intense exercise on the weekends, you could also arrange your week like this:

YOUR SILVER MONTH 1 ROUTINE

MONDAY:	Interval training
TUESDAY:	Strength training
WEDNESDAY:	Moderate cardio
THURSDAY:	Strength training
FRIDAY:	Moderate cardio
SATURDAY:	Easy bike ride
SUNDAY:	Hike with family

As you can see, you have some leeway here, including which days of the week you exercise, how many moderate cardio sessions (one or two), and how many interval sessions (one or two) you do each week. Within the parameters listed, feel free to change it up from week to week, doing different activities on different days, and shifting your focus from less intense (more moderate cardio) to more intense (more interval training), depending on your mood and energy level.

Ready? Let's roll. . . .

MONTH 1
STRENGTH
TRAINING

There are two different strength-training workouts this month, both of which work your entire body in slightly different ways. Do each workout once a week.

Your equipment needs are minimal: a pair of dumbbells or kettlebells, a Physioball (Swiss ball), a TRX suspension trainer (or similar device), and a stopwatch or timepiece with a second hand. *NOTE: If you don't have access to equipment, or are unable to make it to the gym, you can also try the no-equipment options, listed alongside each exercise that involves equipment.*

After your warmup, set up everything you need for each exercise so you can transition easily from one move to the next. Then start your stopwatch and perform as many good-form reps of the first move as you can in 40 seconds. Rest 20 seconds, repeat the same process for the next exercise, and so on. When you've completed all 10, rest for 2 minutes and repeat the cycle one more time—or, if you're feeling particularly energetic, twice—for a total workout time of either 22 or 34 minutes.

You should always be working at or close to your maximum capacity for each 40–second work period. If the set feels too easy, speed up. If your form starts to fall apart, slow down. As you proceed through the month, you'll find you can do more reps of each exercise during each 40–second work period.

WORKOUT #1

BODY-WEIGHT JUMP SQUAT

Place your fingers on the back of your head and pull your elbows back so that they're in line with your body. Perform a body-weight squat until your thighs are parallel to the floor, then explosively jump as high as you can (imagine you're pushing the floor away from you as you leap). When you land, immediately squat and jump again. Hold dumbbells at your side to make it more challenging.

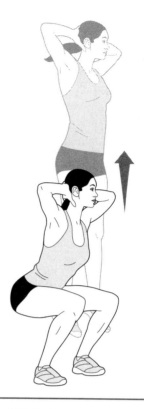

40-SECOND OUT-AND-BACK SPRINT

This is pretty simple: Sprint for 20 seconds in one direction, then turn around and sprint back to start (outdoors). You can also do this indoors on a treadmill by turning up the speed to sprint level and going for 40 seconds.

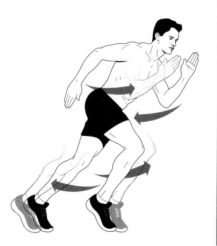

NO-ROOM OR NO-TREADMILL OPTION: SPLIT JUMP

Stand in a staggered stance, your left foot in front of your right. Lower your body as far as you can. Quickly switch directions and jump with enough force to propel both feet off the floor. While in the air, scissor-kick your legs so you land with the opposite leg forward. Repeat, alternating back and forth with each repetition.

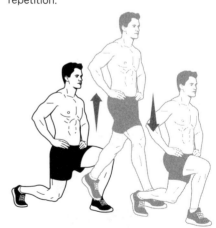

T-PUSHUP

Set yourself in pushup position with your feet hip-width apart. Your hands should be slightly wider than shoulder-width apart. Lower your body to the floor. As you push yourself back up, in one fluid motion, rotate the right side of your body upward as you lift your right arm so that it's extended above your right shoulder (your arms should form a T with your body). Lower your arm and repeat, this time performing the move to your left.

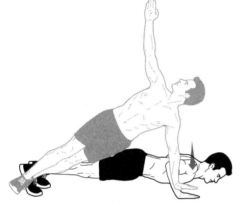

WIDE-STANCE PLANK WITH OPPOSITE ARM AND LEG LIFT

• Start to get in the pushup position, but bend your elbows and rest your weight on your forearms instead of on your hands. Your body should form a straight line from your shoulders to your ankles. Move your feet out wider than your shoulders.

• Brace your core by contracting your abs as if you're about to be punched in the gut. Now raise your left foot and right arm off the floor and hold. Halfway through the prescribed time, switch to the other arm and leg.

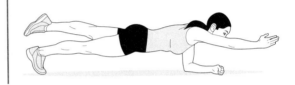

STEP-UP

Stand in front of a bench or step and place your right foot firmly on the step. Press your heel into the step and push your body up until your right leg is straight. Pause for a second, then lower your body back down until your left foot touches the floor, then repeat. Halfway through the time allotted, switch feet.

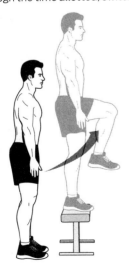

INVERTED ROW

Lie on your back under a bar and grab the bar with an overhand, shoulder-width grip. The bar should be set high enough to allow your shoulders to be just off the ground when your arms are fully straight. Your body should form a straight line from your ankles to your head. Initiate movement by pulling your shoulder blades back, then continue the pull with your arms to lift your chest to the bar. Pause, then slowly lower your body back to the starting position. Keep your body rigid the entire movement and try to keep your wrists straight.

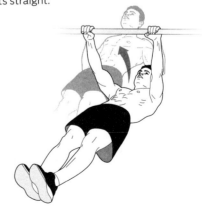

WORKOUT #1—*Continued*

COBRA (NO-EQUIPMENT OPTION)
• Lie facedown on the floor with your legs straight and your arms next to your sides, palms down.

• Contract your glutes and the muscles of your lower back, and raise your head, chest, arms, and legs off the floor.

• Simultaneously rotate your arms so that your thumbs point toward the ceiling. At this time, your hips should be the only parts of your body touching the floor. Hold this position for the prescribed time.

NOTE: If you can't hold it for the entire time, hold for 5 to 10 seconds, rest for 5, and repeat as many times as needed. If the exercise is too easy, you can hold light dumbbells in your hands while you do it.

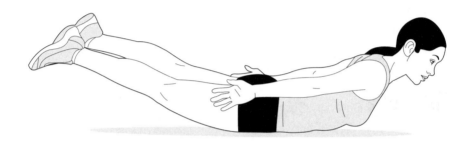

ELBOW-TO-KNEE CRUNCH
Lie faceup with your hips and knees bent 90 degrees so that your lower legs are parallel to the floor. Place your fingers on the sides of your head. Lift your shoulders off the floor as if doing a crunch. Twist your upper body to the left while bringing up your left knee to touch your right elbow. Simultaneously straighten your right leg. Return to the starting position and repeat to the other side.

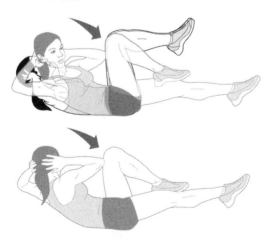

DUMBBELL SHOULDER PRESS
Stand holding a pair of dumbbells just outside your shoulders, with your arms bent and palms facing each other. Set your feet shoulder-width apart and slightly bend your knees. Press the weights upward until your arms are completely straight. Slowly lower the dumbbells back to the starting position. Keep your core braced throughout the movement.

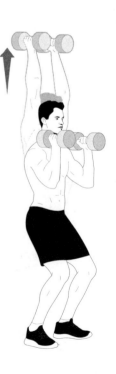

INCHWORM (NO-EQUIPMENT OPTION)

• Stand tall with your legs straight and bend over and touch the floor. Keeping your legs straight, walk your hands forward (if you can't reach the floor with your legs straight, bend your knees just enough so you can. As your flexibility improves, try to straighten them a little more). Keeping your core braced, walk your hands out as far as you can without allowing your hips to sag.

• Then take tiny steps to walk your feet back to your hands. That's 1 repetition. Do 5 forward, and then 5 more in reverse.

SWISS BALL PIKE

Assume pushup position with your arms completely straight, your hands slightly wider than your shoulders. Rest your shins on a Swiss ball. Your body should form a straight line from your head to your ankles. Without bending your knees, roll the Swiss ball toward your body by raising your hips as high as you can. Don't round your lower back. Pause, then return the ball to the starting position by lowering your hips and rolling the ball backward.

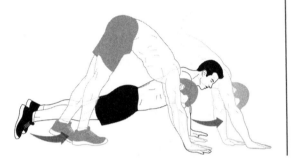

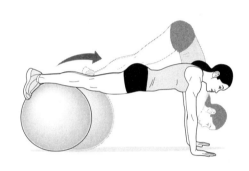

SKATER JUMP

Stand on your right foot with your right knee slightly bent and place your left foot just behind your right ankle. Bend your right knee and lower your body into a partial squat. Then bound to the left by jumping off your right foot. Land on your left foot and bring your right foot behind your left as you reach toward the floor with your right hand. Repeat the move back toward the right, landing on your right foot and left hand. (This exercise mimics the fluid side-to-side movement of a speed skater.)

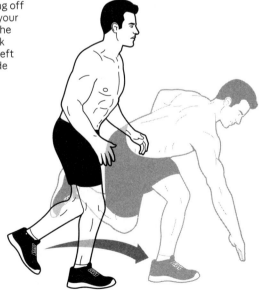

WORKOUT #2

SWING

Take an overhead grip on a dumbbell or kettlebell and assume a shoulder-width-and-a-half stance with your feet pointed slightly outward. Keeping your back straight and your gaze forward, thrust your hips explosively forward and swing the dumbbell or kettlebell up to about eye level, squeezing your glutes hard at the top of the move. Hinging forward at your hip joint and bending your knees slightly, allow the weight to swing down and back between your legs. Repeat for prescribed reps, focusing on the explosive hip-thrust move on each rep.

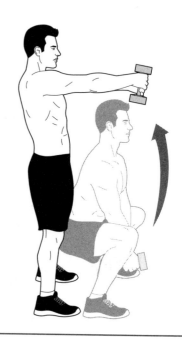

STEP-UP 20 SECONDS PER SIDE

Stand in front of a bench or step and place your right foot firmly on the step. Press your heel into the step and push your body up until your right leg is straight. Pause for a second, then lower your body back down until your left foot touches the floor, then repeat. Halfway through the time allotted, switch feet.

PUSHUP

Get into pushup position using your hands as a base (you can also grip hexagonal dumbbells as your base). Keeping your body straight from your head to your ankles, lower your body until your chest nearly touches the ground. Pause at the bottom and then push yourself back to the starting position as quickly as possible.

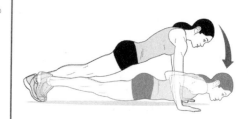

V-UP

Lie faceup on the floor with your legs straight and your arms straight above the top of your head, in line with your body. In one movement, simultaneously lift your torso and legs as if you're trying to touch your toes. Keep your head in line with your body; don't crane your neck. Your legs should be straight and your torso and legs should form a V. Lower your body back to the starting position.

BODY-WEIGHT BULGARIAN SPLIT SQUAT

Stand in a staggered stance, your left foot in front of your right 2 to 3 feet apart. Place just the instep of your back foot on a bench or chair. Pull your shoulders back and brace your core. Lower your body as deeply as you can, keeping your back foot on the bench. Keep your shoulders back and chest up through the movement. Pause, then return to the starting position. Halfway through the prescribed time, switch to the other foot.

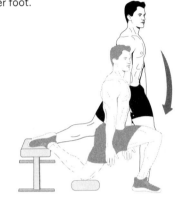

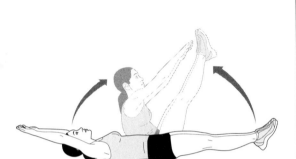

BURPEE (DUMBBELL OPTIONAL)

Stand with your feet shoulder-width apart and arms at your sides. Lower your body into as deep a squat as you can. Now kick your legs backward so that you're in pushup position, then quickly bring your legs back into the squat position. Stand up quickly and jump. That's 1 rep.

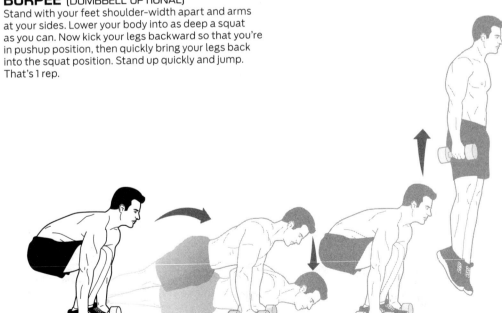

WORKOUT #2—*Continued*

ALTERNATING RENEGADE ROW

Select a pair of medium-weight dumbbells and assume a pushup position, feet shoulder-width apart and hands directly beneath your shoulders, gripping the dumbbell handles for support. Minimizing any rolling or tilting in the hips, shift the entire weight of your upper body onto your left hand and pull the dumbbell in your right hand toward your right hip as if performing a single-arm dumbbell row. Lower the dumbbell to the starting position, shift your weight onto your right hand and repeat on the left side. Alternate sides for sets of 10 to 15 repetitions each side.

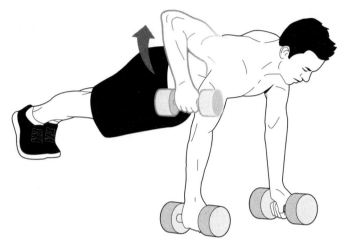

PRONE SWIM

(NO-EQUIPMENT OPTION)

Lie on your stomach with your arms extended overhead and your back arched so your head is off the floor. Keeping your arms straight and your hands off the floor, bring your hands toward your sides as if performing a prone jumping-jack. Return to the starting position. That's 1 rep.

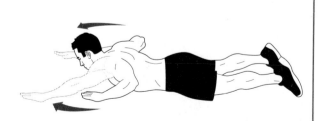

SPLIT JUMP

Stand in a staggered stance, your left foot in front of your right. Lower your body as far as you can. Quickly switch directions and jump with enough force to propel both feet off the floor. While in the air, scissor-kick your legs so you land with the opposite leg forward. Repeat, alternating back and forth with each repetition.

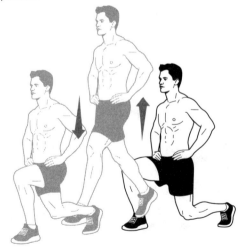

ROLLING SIDE PLANK

Start by performing a side plank with your left side down. Hold for 1 or 2 seconds, then roll your body over onto both elbows—into a traditional plank—and hold for 1 or 2 seconds. Next, roll all the way up onto your right hand so that you're performing a side plank facing the opposite direction. Hold for another second or two. That's 1 repetition. Make sure to move your whole body as a single unit each time you roll.

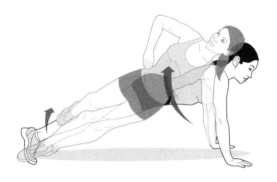

DUMBBELL CHOP

(20 SECONDS PER SIDE)

Grab a dumbbell and hold it with both hands above your right shoulder. Stand with your feet shoulder-width apart. Brace your core and rotate your torso to your right. While keeping your arms straight, swing the dumbbell down and to the outside of your left knee by rotating to the left and bending at your hips. Reverse the movement to return to the start. Halfway through the prescribed time, switch sides.

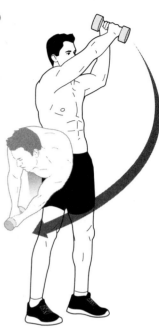

MOUNTAIN CLIMBER

Get in pushup position with your arms straight. This is the starting position. Lift your left foot and raise your knee as close to your chest as you can. Touch the ground with your left foot and then return to the starting position and repeat with your right leg. Go as fast as possible.

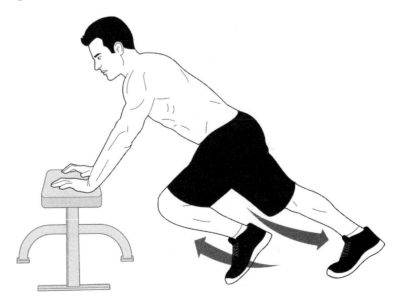

MONTH 1
CARDIO FUN

Since the 1970s, health professionals have recommended exercising at a steady, sustainable pace for 20 minutes or more. I agree with this recommendation—especially if you like doing this type of exercise, and even more if you're an endurance athlete. And this month, you'll still be doing one or two of these types of workouts every week.

However, you're also going to be putting another weapon into your fitness-boosting, fat-blasting arsenal: *interval training.*

In recent years, this type of training—repeated, higher-intensity bouts of exercise performed for shorter periods, and interspersed with periods of rest—has become more popular for general fitness. Rather than simply jogging eight laps around the track, for example, a runner might sprint for half a lap, walk slowly for the other half, and repeat the cycle four to six times. Or you can use a timed approach, running for 30 seconds, resting for 90, and repeating.

There are plenty of benefits to this type of training. It *may* be more effective for burning fat than a longer, slower approach. It may also build—or at least help you maintain—muscle mass in ways that slow training doesn't. Indisputably, it's less time-consuming, and increases speed and power more effectively, than slower training. And people who find

long, slow cardio dull may get a surprising kick out of interval training. Children rarely jog for long periods, but they sprint all the time—because it's fun. You'll probably agree.

Interval training also offers exercisers of all skill levels a ton of options. If you hate running, you can interval train on a bike, in a pool, on an elliptical trainer, or in an exercise room using a jump rope or calisthenics. A beginner can start with a few 10-second bouts of medium effort on a stationary bike, resting 50 seconds after each one. An advanced athlete might do 10 or more 2-minute high-effort sprints on the bike, separated by just 30 seconds of rest. As long as both are working close to their capacity, both will benefit. As you improve or simply tire of one particular approach, you can adjust the duration of the work periods, the duration of the rest periods, and the number of work-rest rounds you perform.

Team-sport athletes can create interval workouts that closely mimic the demands of their chosen sport. If you play touch football or Ultimate Frisbee, for example, you might do repeated 40-yard sprints separated by 1-minute rest periods to approximate the demands of a game.

The downside to formal interval training is that it's fairly advanced—especially if you choose a high-impact activity like running. After you've done interval training for a while, you'll know just how hard to push if they're doing work periods that last 10 seconds, 30 seconds, or 1 minute.

Beginners, on the other hand, will have to guess. So ease into it, and never do these types of workouts more than three times a week on nonconsecutive days.

Below are eight interval-training workouts you can start to experiment with this month, and return to as you continue to reach higher levels of fitness. Repeat the work-rest cycle for the suggested number of rounds.

TABATA

WORK:	20 seconds
REST:	10 seconds
REPS:	6–8
SUGGESTED EXERCISES:	Running, jumping rope, calisthenics

Named for Japanese exercise physiologist Izumi Tabata, this method uses brief work periods followed by even shorter rest periods. Repeat six to eight times for a very brief, but very challenging high-intensity workout. Beginners, remember to go easy on this one—it's a bear. Advanced folks, go for it, but be ready for a serious challenge. This one was designed to take Olympic-caliber speed skaters to the next level.

TWO-ON, TWO-OFF

WORK:	2 minutes
REST:	2 minutes
REPS:	3–4
SUGGESTED EXERCISES:	Running, cycling, jumping rope, calisthenics

Twelve or sixteen minutes will be all the workout you need. Two minutes—roughly the amount of time that world-class runners can complete the half-mile—is a particularly challenging interval. It's not quite a sprint and not quite a jog. If you're pressed for time at the gym, this is a good option to do on an elliptical trainer or any piece of cardio equipment.

TIME LADDER

WORK:	1, 2, 3, then 4 minutes
REST:	1, 2, 3, then 4 minutes
REPS:	4 (once up the ladder) or 8 (once up, then down the ladder)
SUGGESTED EXERCISES:	Cycling, cardio machines

This one comes recommended by famed triathlon coach Joe Friel, author of *The Triathlete's Training Bible*, and is a great one to do on a bike—just make sure you're on a fairly flat, secluded road that's largely free of stoplights. After a warmup, go all-out for a minute, then easy for a minute; then all-out for 2 minutes, easy for 2, and so on, up to a 4-minute work set. If you've got the time and energy, work your way back down the ladder for a workout totaling 40 minutes. You can also invert the workout, starting and finishing with the 4-minute work sets.

THE QUARTER HORSE

WORK:	1 minute
REST:	2 minutes
REPS:	3–8
SUGGESTED EXERCISES:	Running, cardio machines

This might be the simplest break-in interval program of them all. If you're running on a track, note the distance you covered in the first minute-long interval, and try to match or exceed it in subsequent rounds. If your distance suddenly drops off, hang it up for the day—you've pushed a little too hard.

WIND-SPRINT FUN

WORK:	30 seconds
REST:	150 seconds (2:30)
REPS:	4–8
SUGGESTED EXERCISES:	Running, treadmill running, cardio machines

Wind sprints sneak up on you: 30 seconds, even at a hard pace, doesn't seem too bad at first, especially when you're resting a full 2.5 minutes between sets. Then, suddenly, it does. It *really* does. The long rest periods allow you to work at close to your maximum with each effort—making this workout a little more like a strength workout than a cardio workout.

THE CLOCK WATCHER

WORK:	variable
REST:	variable
REPS:	variable
SUGGESTED EXERCISES:	Swimming

This is a system used quite effectively by swimmers. Choose a time interval—say, 2 minutes—and a distance—say, 50 yards. Note the time you begin your swim. On each round, complete the 50-yard distance and rest for the remainder of your 2-minute interval. Repeat for reps—say, four if you're just starting out. Go hard and you get more rest. Go slower and you'll get less. Over time you'll learn to choose an interval that matches your fitness level.

Now you know what the big, stopwatch-style clock next to the pool is for and why the guys in goggles and swim caps are staring at it all the time.

SHUTTLE RUN

WORK:	30 seconds
REST:	1 minute
REPS:	2–5
SUGGESTED EXERCISES:	Running

Team-sports players will be familiar with this drill: Place two objects (cones work well) 10 to 20 yards apart on a flat, grassy field. Run back and forth between them for 30 seconds, trying to change directions as fast as you can when you reach the cones. Even if you never reach your top sprint speed, the change of direction makes this one a serious challenge, and great for building sports-specific quickness and agility.

FARMER'S CARRY

WORK:	2 minutes
REST:	1 minute
REPS:	2–4
SUGGESTED EXERCISES:	Brisk walking

In the classic version, you grab a heavy dumbbell in each hand and walk as far as you can without putting them down. But there are plenty of alternatives from easy to super-advanced: Hold a weight plate or a medicine ball. Carry one dumbbell only. Carry the implement at or above shoulder height. Use a StepMill (the escalator-like cardio machine) or a treadmill, inclined or flat. Walk up and down actual stairs. Carry a friend, piggy-back or fireman style, then let them carry you, on the flat or up a hill, or up the stairs. Challenging but safe, the farmer's carry is one of the most versatile, effective, and rarely used exercises there is, and perfect for interval training.

The Essential Home Gym
(FOR UNDER $400!)

Commercial gyms give you the impression that getting fit requires lots of bulky equipment. But the good old-fashioned chinup gives your biceps a better workout than the seated curl machine, and a quick run up a steep hill is far better for your quads than the leg extension device.

You just don't need a whole lot of stuff to get exceptionally fit—and what you *do* need certainly doesn't need to take up your whole living room—or your whole budget. If you've got $400, spend it on these six items. They're all the home gym you'll ever need:

1. Suspension Trainer (TRX or Equivalent): The suspension trainer is one of those "shoulda thought of that" fitness tools that's gained popularity in the last couple of years. Essentially, it's a couple of nylon straps with handles that you can attach to something elevated (a door frame or a tree branch) and use to perform dozens of variations on novel and classic body-weight strength-training moves. It's very useful for rows and core training, and you can't beat it for convenience: the TRX rolls up into a 2-pound, grapefruit-size mesh bag. **Cost: $200**

2. Jump Rope: Another cardio standby that you can toss in a suitcase or gym bag for a quick, do-anywhere workout. Jumping rope is a terrific, full-body exercise—preferable, in my opinion, to the workout you get on most cardio machines. You'll also develop timing, hand-eye coordination, and an appreciation for the fitness levels of both champion boxers and 8-year-old girls. I like the fast-moving, inexpensive plastic kind, but was recently introduced to a 2-inch-thick, 7-foot-long model—a real beast and a great option if you want an advanced upper-body challenge. **Cost: Plastic—$10; Thick—$40**

3. Chinup Bar: For anyone trying to get leaner, stronger, and more athletic, some form of chinup should be a staple. The chinup builds *relative strength,* or the ability to move your body through space quickly and easily, and works muscles that help to improve the slouching, rounded-forward posture most of us are stuck in for 8 or more hours a day. Plus, being able to bang out eight or more chinups is a mark of serious fitness, and an accomplishment to strive for.

If you buy your own chinup bar, install it in a centrally located doorway, and do a single jump-and-pull chinup every time you pass the bar. Pretty soon you'll be chinning with the best of them.

Get the kind that fits easily over a doorframe without bolts or screws. **Cost: $50**

4. Kettlebell: You've probably seen these thick-handled, odd-shaped weights cropping up on fitness shows and lurking in corners at your local gym. If you're going to buy a single weighted implement for home use, get one of these before investing in costly dumbbells and clunky, space-sucking barbells. Press it, lift it off the ground, swing it, carry it. Be creative.

If you get ambitious, you can learn the handful of simple moves taught by the kettlebell experts—swings, snatches, cleans, and get-ups. After a while you'll wonder why people ever use anything else. Get a weight you can press overhead a few times with one hand. When that gets too easy, get the next size up. **Cost: around $60 (varies depending on weight)**

5. Foam Roller: Who knew that industrial Styrofoam could be such an effective massage tool? Hurts so good. For maintaining healthy and pain-free movement, this might be the best $30 to $45 you'll ever spend. **Cost: $30**

6. Medicine Ball: Some fitness pros use the terms "strength" and "power" interchangeably, but they're really two different things. *Strength* refers to your ability to move a weight; *power* refers to your ability to move that weight *fast*. Squatting requires strength; jumping requires power.

We lose power as we age, even faster than we lose strength—that's one of the reasons older people have a hard time catching themselves when they fall. To combat this, a good workout program should always include some type of fast, powerful movement.

Plyometrics—jumping of various kinds—takes care of the power in the lower body. The medicine ball, which you can throw, smash, and slam in a variety of tension-relieving ways, is your go-to tool for upper-body power. Get the kind that bounces, and don't be fooled into thinking heavier is better. Even muscle-heads will get all the workout they need out of 10 to 12 pounds. **Cost: $25**

MONTH 2

For your second month on the Silver-Level training program (and fifth month overall, if you started out at Bronze Level), you'll be kicking things up a notch once again, doing slightly more difficult strength-training workouts three times a week, rather than twice.

You'll probably notice that something significant seems to happen when you add that third weekly strength-training session into the mix, especially since you've built up to it for at least a month. Strength gains will come more quickly. You'll burn more fat, build more muscle. I've seen it happen over and over: Three times a week is the "Goldilocks" level for most people, just the right amount of stimulation and rest to promote optimal gains.

At the same time, however, it's even more important this month that you take a close look at your diet and arrange your food consumption to support and enhance your exercise efforts. The better and cleaner your diet, the better you will feel, and stronger you'll get, and the better your results will be.

Once again, your foam-rolling and dynamic warmups will stay the same as in previous months (three times a week and before every hard workout, respectively). You'll also stick with interval training and moderate cardio workouts, as well as easy walks at least twice a week—and

more often if you can fit them in. And keep the NEAT going as well: Break up periods of sitting by taking microbreaks every 20 minutes or so, and by walking as much as possible throughout your day.

A sample week of training might look like this:

YOUR SILVER MONTH 2 ROUTINE	
MONDAY:	Strength training
TUESDAY:	Moderate cardio or interval training
WEDNESDAY:	Strength cardio
THURSDAY:	Easy walk
FRIDAY:	Strength training
SATURDAY:	Interval training or moderate cardio
SUNDAY:	Easy walk

Again this month, you'll be working on the clock—doing as many good-form reps as you can for the allotted time period. You'll do each workout—A, B, and C—once a week on nonconsecutive days—say, Monday, Wednesday, and Friday, repeating the cycle about four times throughout the month. If you miss a workout, pick up where you left off: There's nothing magical about doing workout A first in the week, B second, and so on. Equipment needs are still minimal, though you might consider joining a gym, or investing in some heavier kettlebells or dumbbells as you progress with the program.

These three workouts consist of a lot of *plyometric* exercises: movements that require explosive force, such as jumps and throwing movements. These are among my favorite types of strength-training moves. They're great for building athletic performance, since most sports require speed and acceleration, but they're also essential for maintaining quality of life in older adults as well. Plyometrics help preserve bone density, as well as suppleness and elasticity through the fascial tissue—all essential for healthy movement and mobility. And maintaining power—or the ability to move fast—is one of the first qualities we lose as we age. This age-related loss of power accounts for many of the injuries that older adults suffer when they fall.

The other reason I like plyometrics is that—I'll go ahead and admit this here—they never get easy. For anyone. Forty-five seconds of squat jumps, for example, is hard for any-one. I'm all for training with weights (we'll do more of that when you graduate to the Gold Level), but for now, focus on moving as fast and powerfully as you can through those explosive moves while maintaining good form: I promise you'll get a great workout, however advanced you are.

Do as many reps of each movement as you can in 45 seconds; then rest for 15 seconds and move to the next exercise. When you've completed all 10 moves, rest for 2 minutes and cycle through all 10 moves one—or if you're feeling spry—two more times, for a total of two or three times through the routine, and a total workout time of 22 or 34 minutes.

These workouts are tough—harder exercises, more work, less rest. But by now you should be ready for the extra challenge. Good luck!

WORKOUT A

THRUSTER

Assume an athletic stance, feet parallel and slightly wider than shoulder width, holding two equally-weighted dumbbells or kettlebells at shoulder height, palms facing toward each other. Keeping your chest up, gaze forward, and your back straight, squat down until the tops of your thighs are parallel to the floor, or as far as you can without losing the natural arch in your lower back. Quickly reverse the movement, pressing the weight explosively overhead when you reach the standing position. Lower the weights back to shoulder height. That's 1 rep.

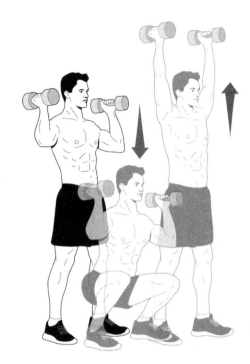

TRX ROW

Hold a TRX handle in each hand and back away until you feel tension in the straps. Your body should form a 45- to 60-degree angle to the floor (the deeper the angle, the harder the exercise), and your arms should be parallel to the floor, palms down. Pull your body toward the anchor point by bringing the handles to the sides of your chest as you rotate your palms inward. Your elbows should be at 45 degrees. Pause and return to the starting position.

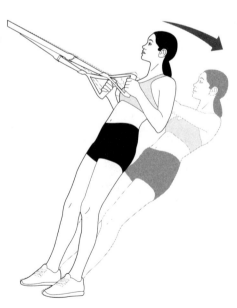

BURPEE WITH JUMP (DUMBBELLS OPTIONAL)

Stand with your feet shoulder-width apart and arms at your sides. Lower your body into as deep a squat as you can. Now kick your legs backward so that you're in pushup position, then quickly bring your legs back into the squat position. Stand up quickly and jump. That's 1 rep.

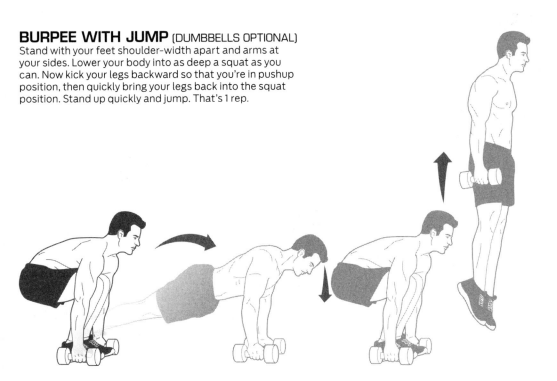

SWISS BALL ROLLOUT

Kneel in front of a Swiss ball and place your forearms and fists on the ball. Your lower back should be naturally arched and your elbows bent about 90 degrees. While keeping your core braced, slowly roll the ball forward, straightening your arms and extending your body as far as you can without allowing your lower back to "collapse." Pause, then use your abdominal muscles to pull the ball back to your knees.

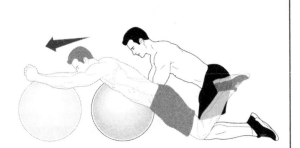

BODY-WEIGHT BULGARIAN SPLIT SQUAT

Stand in a staggered stance, your left foot in front of your right 2 to 3 feet apart. Place just the instep of your back foot on a bench or chair. Pull your shoulders back and brace your core. Lower your body as deeply as you can, keeping your back foot on the bench. Keep your shoulders back and chest up through the movement. Pause, then return to the starting position. Halfway through the prescribed time, switch to the other foot.

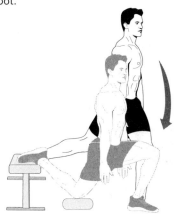

WORKOUT A—*Continued*

PUSHUP
Get into pushup position with your hands shoulder-width apart. Keeping your body straight from your head to your ankles, lower your body until your chest nearly touches the floor. Pause at the bottom and then push yourself back to the starting position as quickly as possible.

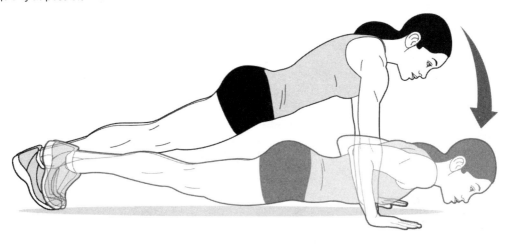

NO-ROOM OR NO-TREADMILL OPTION: SPLIT JUMP
Stand in a staggered stance, your left foot in front of your right. Lower your body as far as you can. Quickly switch directions and jump with enough force to propel both feet off the floor. While in the air, scissor-kick your legs so you land with the opposite leg forward. Repeat, alternating back and forth with each repetition.

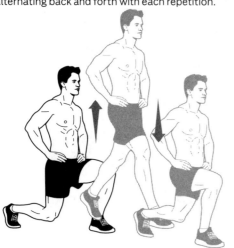

45-SECOND OUT-AND-BACK SPRINT
This is pretty simple: Sprint for 22 seconds in one direction, then turn around and sprint back to start (outdoors). You can also do this indoors on a treadmill by turning up the speed to sprint level and going for 45 seconds.

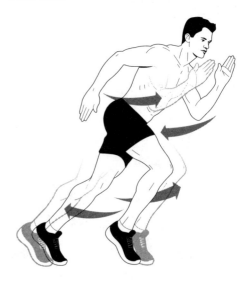

V-UP

Lie faceup on the floor with your legs straight and your arms straight above the top of your head, in line with your body. In one movement, simultaneously lift your torso and legs as if you're trying to touch your toes. Keep your head in line with your body; don't crane your neck. Your legs should be straight and your torso and legs should form a V. Lower your body back to the starting position.

MOUNTAIN CLIMBER

Get in pushup position with your arms straight. This is the starting position. Lift your left foot and raise your knee as close to your chest as you can. Touch the ground with your left foot and then return to the starting position and repeat with your right leg. Go as fast as possible.

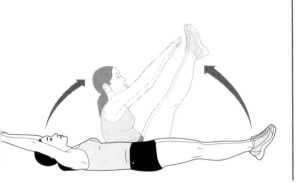

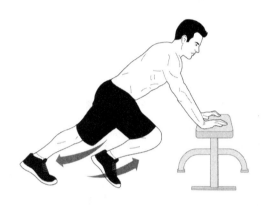

TURKISH GET-UP

Lie faceup with your legs straight. Hold a dumbbell in your left hand with your arm straight above you. Don't take your eyes off the dumbbell at any time. Roll onto your right side and prop yourself up on your right elbow. Place your left foot flat on the floor, then push yourself into a position with your right knee down and your left foot still flat on the floor. Simply stand up, while keeping your arm straight and the dumbbell above you at all times. Once standing, reverse the movement to return to the starting position. Halfway through the prescribed time, switch hands.

WORKOUT B

SQUAT JUMP
Holding you hands in front of your chest, perform a body-weight squat until your thighs are parallel to the floor, then explosively jump as high as you can (imagine you're pushing the floor away from you as you leap). When you land, immediately squat and jump again. Hold dumbbells at your side to make it more challenging.

PULLUP
Grab the pullup bar with a shoulder-width, overhand grip. Hang at arm's length. Cross your ankles behind you. You should return to this position—known as a dead hang—each time you lower your body back down. Squeeze your shoulder blades together as you pull your chest to the bar. Once the top of your chest touches the bar, pause, then slowly lower your body back to a dead hang.

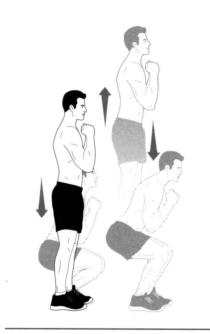

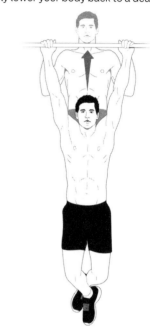

WIDE-STANCE PLANK WITH OPPOSITE ARM AND LEG LIFT
• Start to get in the pushup position, but bend your elbows and rest your weight on your forearms instead of on your hands. Your body should form a straight line from your shoulders to your ankles. Move your feet out wider than your shoulders.

• Brace your core by contracting your abs as if you're about to be punched in the gut. Now raise your left foot and right arm off the floor and hold. Halfway through the prescribed time, switch to the other arm and leg.

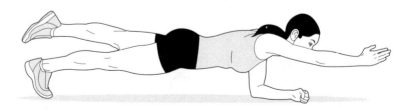

JUMP ROPE
45 seconds

WALKING LUNGE (DUMBBELLS OPTIONAL)

• Perform a lunge, but instead of pushing your body backward to the starting position, rise up and bring your back foot forward so that you move forward (as if you're walking) a step with every rep. Alternate the leg you step forward with each time.

• Halfway through your prescribed time, perform backward walking lunges to return to your starting point.

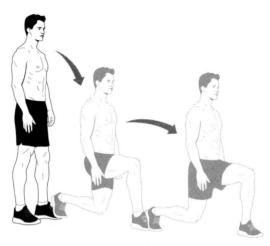

DUMBBELL PUSH PRESS

Stand holding a pair of dumbbells just outside your shoulders, with your arms bent and palms facing each other. Stand with your feet shoulder-width apart and knees slightly bent. Dip your knees and explosively push up with your legs as you press the weights straight over your shoulders. Lower the dumbbells back to the starting position and repeat.

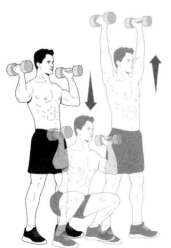

SWISS BALL PIKE

Assume pushup position with your arms completely straight, your hands slightly wider than your shoulders. Rest your shins on a Swiss ball. Your body should form a straight line from your head to your ankles. Without bending your knees, roll the Swiss ball toward your body by raising your hips as high as you can. Don't round your lower back. Pause, then return the ball to the starting position by lowering your hips and rolling the ball backward.

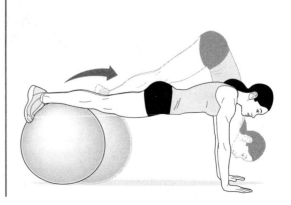

WORKOUT B—*Continued*

SKATER JUMP

Stand on your right foot with your right knee slightly bent, and place your left foot just behind your right ankle. Bend your right knee and lower your body into a partial squat. Then bound to the left by jumping off your right foot. Land on your left foot and bring your right foot behind your left as you reach toward the floor with your right hand. Repeat the move back toward the right, landing on your right foot and left hand. (This exercise mimics the fluid side-to-side movement of a speed skater.)

DUMBBELL/KETTLEBELL STRAIGHT-LEG DEADLIFT TO ROW

Let a pair of dumbbells (or kettlebells) hang at arm's length in front of your hips. Your palms should face your thighs. Bend at your hips and lower your torso into a bent-over position. Keep your lower back naturally arched. Pull the weights to the sides of your torso (without moving your torso). Pause, then lower the weights and return to the standing position.

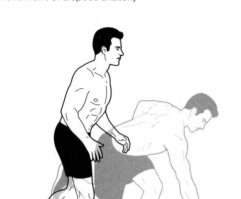

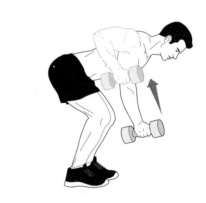

FEET-ELEVATED PUSHUP

Get into pushup position using your hands as a base (you can also grip hexagonal dumbbells as your base). Place your feet on a step or bench to elevate them. Keeping your body straight from your head to your ankles, lower your body until your chest nearly touches the ground. Pause at the bottom and then push yourself back to the starting position as quickly as possible.

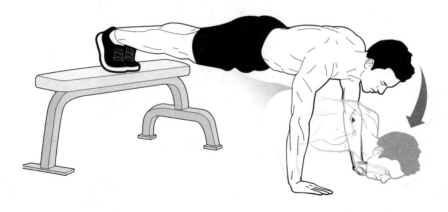

WORKOUT C

SINGLE-ARM DUMBBELL/ KETTLEBELL SWING

Hold a dumbbell (or kettlebell) at arm's length in front of your waist. Without rounding your lower back, bend at your hips and knees and swing the dumbbell between your legs. Keeping your arm straight, thrust your hips forward and swing the dumbbell to shoulder level as you rise to a standing position. Swing the weight back and forth. Halfway through your time, switch arms.

RENEGADE ROW

Select a pair of medium-weight dumbbells and assume a pushup position, feet shoulder-width apart and hands directly beneath your shoulders, gripping the dumbbell handles for support. Minimizing any rolling or tilting in the hips, shift the entire weight of your upper body onto your left hand and pull the dumbbell in your right hand toward your right hip as if performing a single-arm dumbbell row. Lower the dumbbell to the starting position, shift your weight onto your right hand and repeat on the left side. Alternate sides for sets of 10 to 15 repetitions each side.

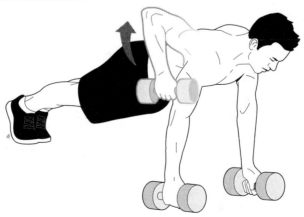

WORKOUT C—*Continued*

LYING BALL PASS, HANDS TO FEET

Lie on your back, holding a small- to medium-size Swiss ball in your hands directly over your chest. Forcefully bracing your core and pressing your lower back toward the floor, lift your legs until they are pointed directly toward the ceiling. With your head relaxed on the floor, transfer the ball from your hands to your legs, gripping it with your lower legs and feet. Keeping your thighs pointed straight up, bend your knees and lower the ball until it is a couple of inches from the floor. As you lower your legs, simultaneously reach and stretch your arms toward the floor over your head, keeping them parallel. Keeping your lower back pressed toward the floor, raise your arms and legs until they are above your torso again, and transfer the ball from your legs to your hands. Lower your hands and feet toward the floor again, this time holding the ball with your hands. Bring the arms and legs back to the starting position and transfer the ball back to your feet. Count 1 rep each time you transfer the ball.

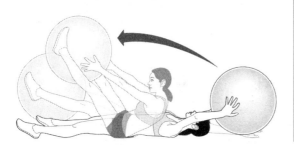

MOUNTAIN CLIMBER

Get in pushup position with your arms straight. This is the starting position. Lift your left foot and raise your knee as close to your chest as you can. Touch the ground with your left foot and then return to the starting position and repeat with your right leg. Go as fast as possible.

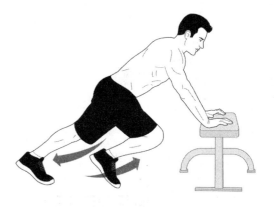

STEP-UP

(DUMBBELLS OPTIONAL)

Stand in front of a bench or step and place your right foot firmly on the step (to make this exercise more challenging, hold a pair of dumbbells at your sides). Press your heel into the step and push your body up until your right leg is straight. Pause for a second, then lower your body back down until your left foot touches the floor, then repeat. Halfway through the time allotted, switch feet.

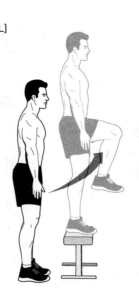

ISO-EXPLOSIVE PUSHUP

Assume the pushup position. Bend your elbows and lower your body until your chest nearly touches the floor. Pause 5 seconds in the down position. Then press yourself up so forcefully that your hands leave the floor. If you need to make this exercise easier, brace your hands on an elevated base like a step or bench.

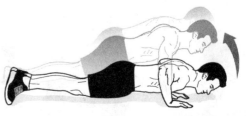

NOTE: This 5-second pause technique eliminates all the elasticity in your muscles, which allows you to activate a maximum number of fast-twitch muscle fibers. These are the fibers with the greatest potential for size and strength gains.

SUICIDES (SHUTTLE RUN)

Sprint five paces, touch the ground, then return to your starting point and touch the ground. Without stopping, now sprint 10 paces, touch the ground, then return to your starting point and touch the ground. Halfway through the prescribed time, start working back down the distance ladder (15 paces, 10 paces, 5 paces, etc.).

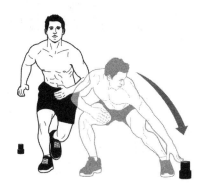

SPLIT JUMP

(NO-ROOM OR NO-TREADMILL OPTION)

Stand in a staggered stance, your left foot in front of your right. Lower your body as far as you can. Quickly switch directions and jump with enough force to propel both feet off the floor. While in the air, scissor-kick your legs so you land with the opposite leg forward. Repeat, alternating back and forth with each repetition.

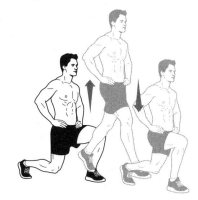

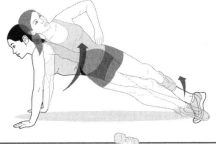

ROLLING SIDE PLANK

Start by performing a side plank with your right side down. Hold for 1 or 2 seconds, then roll your body over—into a traditional pushup position—and hold for 1 or 2 seconds. Next, roll all the way up onto your left hand so that you're performing a side plank facing the opposite direction. Hold for another second or two. That's 1 repetition. Make sure to move your whole body as a single unit each time you roll.

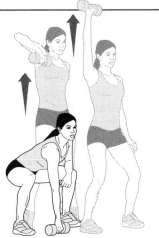

SINGLE-ARM DUMBBELL/ KETTLEBELL SNATCH

Grab a dumbbell (or kettlebell) with an overhand grip. With your feet slightly wider than shoulder-width apart, bend at your hips and knees to squat down until the weight is centered between your feet, your arm straight. Your lower back should be slightly arched. In a single movement, bend your arm, raise your elbow as high as you can, and try to throw the dumbbell at the ceiling (without letting go of it). Keep the dumbbell as close to your body as possible at all times. You should be thrusting the dumbbell upward so forcefully that you rise up on your toes. Allow your forearm to rotate up and back from the momentum of the lift, until your arm is straight and your palm is facing forward. Pull your body under the weight. That's 1 rep. Halfway through the prescribed time, switch arms.

SILVER
MONTH 3

This month, your training schedule will consist of two or three strength-training sessions per week, done on nonconsecutive days (such as Monday, Wednesday, and Friday). On two or three *other* days, you'll do either a brief interval-style workout *or* a slightly longer medium-intensity session (as in previous months). On the remaining days of the week, you'll take an easy 30- to 40-minute walk, hike, bike ride, or swim.

You'll continue to foam-roll, three times a week, and to do a dynamic warmup before all of your tougher workouts. Refer back to the last chapter for these workouts.

Sound complicated? Here's a recap:

YOUR SILVER MONTH 3 ROUTINE	
STRENGTH TRAINING:	2 or 3 times a week
INTERVAL TRAINING:	1 to 3 times a week
MODERATE CARDIO:	0 to 3 times a week
EASY WALK/ RECOVERY DAY:	1 or 2 times a week

You can mix and match on any given week, emphasizing strength training one week, interval training the next. You just want to make sure that:

1. You're always doing something every day.

2. You're never doing the same type of workout 2 days in a row.

So a week of training might look like this:

YOUR SILVER MONTH 3 ROUTINE	
MONDAY:	Foam rolling, dynamic stretching, strength training
TUESDAY:	Dynamic stretching, moderate-intensity cardio
WEDNESDAY:	Foam rolling, dynamic stretching, strength training
THURSDAY:	Easy walk
FRIDAY:	Foam rolling, dynamic stretching, strength training
SATURDAY:	Dynamic stretching, interval training
SUNDAY:	Easy walk

What's with all the choices? Well, my Silver-Level friend, now that you're in your 6th month of exercising regularly, you can start to make some decisions about the types of exercise that best suit you and your goals. If you're interested in building the maximum amount of functional strength and muscle, stick with the three-times-a-week plan that you started last month. If you like interval work, longer-distance work, or if the endurance-event bug is starting to gnaw at you, do more of those workouts. Or you can actually start to switch it up, week to week, depending on your mood, within the parameters listed above.

We'll raise the intensity this month, so keep an eye on your aches and pains. Soreness is fine, but it should dissipate after the first week or so. Interval and strength-training workouts are the ones most likely to make you sore, so if you're in pain, ease off on the intensity or frequency of those workouts.

Even at this phase, none of these workouts should take you more than about 40 minutes, warmups included—unless you decide to walk longer or spend another few minutes on your weight workout.

SILVER
MONTH 3
STRENGTH
TRAINING

This month, you'll strength train either twice or three times a week. If you choose to strength train three times, do the following workouts in order on nonconsecutive days. If you do two workouts a week, start with workouts one and two on the first week and pick up the cycle where you left off in the weeks that follow. So if you do workouts one and two the first week, you'll do workouts three and one the following week, two and three the next, and so on. Keep it up for the entire month, and feel free to switch it up week-to-week.

Each workout is arranged into three circuits. Perform as many reps as you can of each exercise in 50 seconds. Rest for 10 seconds before moving on to the next exercise in the sequence. Perform one circuit of the first three movements, then three or four circuits each of the next two groups of exercises, resting as indicated.

I'm not going to lie; these are seriously taxing workouts. The first time you do each workout, pace yourself so you get the hang of what's coming. In subsequent weeks, feel free to turn up the heat—and the volume—by going harder and faster, and by doing more cycles through each round of exercises.

WORKOUT #1: CIRCUIT ONE

CYCLES:
One or two times through the circuit

V-UP

Lie faceup on the floor with your legs straight and your arms straight above the top of your head, in line with your body. In one movement, simultaneously lift your torso and legs as if you're trying to touch your toes. Keep your head in line with your body; don't crane your neck. Your legs should be straight and your torso and legs should form a V. Lower your body back to the starting position.

WIDE-STANCE PLANK WITH OPPOSITE ARM AND LEG LIFT

• Start to get in the pushup position, but bend your elbows and rest your weight on your forearms instead of on your hands. Your body should form a straight line from your shoulders to your ankles. Move your feet out wider than your shoulders.

• Brace your core by contracting your abs as if you're about to be punched in the gut. Now raise your left foot and right arm off the floor and hold. Halfway through the prescribed time, switch to the other arm and leg.

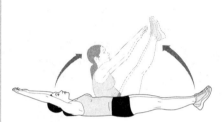

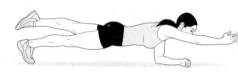

SWISS BALL ALTERNATING TOE TOUCHDOWN

• Assume a pushup position with the tops of your feet elevated on a medium-size Swiss ball. Make sure you body forms a straight line: your head and neck in line with your spine, and your shoulders over your hands.

• Keeping the upper body as motionless as possible and your knees straight, lift your right leg a few inches off the Swiss ball. Extend your right leg to the right of the ball and lower it slowly, tapping the floor with your toes at the bottom of the movement. Slowly lift your right leg back up to rest on top of the ball. Repeat the movement with your left leg, and alternate sides for a total of up to 15 reps on each side. Perform 2 to 3 sets.

• Rest 2 minutes.

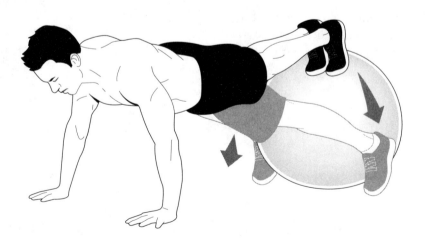

WORKOUT #1: CIRCUIT TWO

THRUSTER

Assume an athletic
stance, feet parallel and
slightly wider than
shoulder width, holding
two equally-weighted
dumbbells or kettlebells
at shoulder height, palms
facing toward each other.
Keeping your chest up,
gaze forward, and your
back straight, squat
down until the tops of
your thighs are parallel
to the floor, or as far as
you can without losing
the natural arch in your
lower back. Quickly
reverse the movement,
pressing the weight
explosively overhead
when you reach the
standing position.
Lower the weights back
to shoulder height.
That's 1 rep.

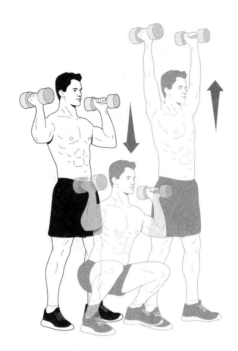

TRX ROW

Hold a TRX handle in each
hand and back away until
you feel tension in the
straps. Your body should
form a 45- to 60-degree
angle to the floor (the
deeper the angle, the
harder the exercise), and
your arms should be parallel to the floor, palms
down. Pull your body
toward the anchor point by
bringing the handles to the
sides of your chest as you
rotate your palms inward.
Your elbows should be at
45 degrees. Pause, and
then return to the starting
position.

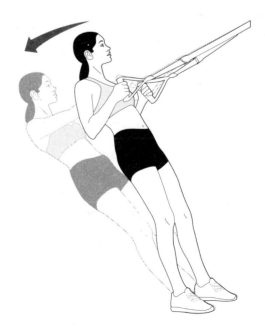

WORKOUT #1 CIRCUIT TWO—*Continued*

REVERSE LUNGE (DUMBBELLS OPTIONAL)
Stand tall with your feet shoulder-width apart. Step backward with your left leg and slowly lower your body until your front knee is bent at least 90 degrees. Your rear knee should nearly touch the floor. Pause, then push yourself to the starting position as quickly as you can. Alternate legs for the prescribed time.

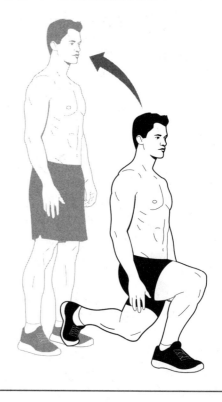

TRX PUSHUP
• Place both feet in the foot cradles of a TRX (the higher the cradles are set, the more challenging the exercise). Get into pushup position. Perform a pushup by lowering your body until your chest is just above the floor. Pause, then press back up.

• Rest 2 minutes.

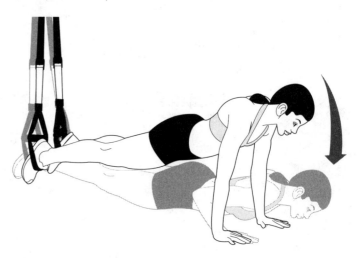

WORKOUT #1: CIRCUIT THREE

CYCLES:
Two to four times through the circuit

BURPEE (WITH PUSHUP AND JUMP)

Stand with your feet shoulder-width apart and arms at your sides. Lower your body into as deep a squat as you can. Now kick your legs backward so that you're in pushup position. Do a pushup, then quickly bring your legs back into the squat position. Stand up quickly and jump. That's 1 rep. (Dumbbells optional, either as a base or to be held throughout entire exercise.)

INVERTED SHOULDER PRESS

• Assume a pushup position, but place your feet on a bench or chair and push your hips up so that your torso is nearly perpendicular to the floor. Your hands should be slightly wider than your shoulders, and your arms should be straight.

• Without changing your body posture, lower your body until your head nearly touches the floor. Pause, then return to the starting position by pushing your body back up until your arms are straight.

NOTE: While the inverted shoulder press is technically a pushup, the tweak to your form shifts more of the workload to your shoulders and triceps, reducing the demand on your chest.

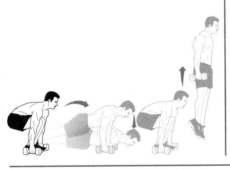

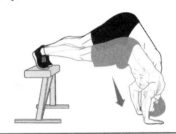

JUMP SQUAT

Perform a body-weight squat until your thighs are parallel to the floor, then explosively jump as high as you can (imagine you're pushing the floor away from you as you leap). When you land, immediately squat and jump again. Hold dumbbells at your side to make it more challenging.

DUMBBELL BICEPS CURL

Grab a pair of dumbbells and let them hang at arm's length next to your sides. Turn your arms so your palms face forward. Without moving your upper arms, bend your elbows and curl the dumbbells as close to your shoulders as you can. Pause, then slowly lower the weights back to the starting position so your arms are straight.

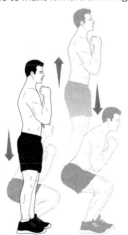

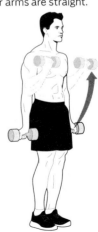

WORKOUT #2: CIRCUIT ONE

CYCLES:
One or two times through the circuit

SIDE PLANK WITH TOP LEG RAISE

(25 SECONDS PER SIDE)
Lie on your side and use your forearm to support your body. One ankle should be on top of the other. Raise your hips until your body forms a straight line from shoulder to ankles. Now lift your top leg until it's a foot to 18 inches above the bottom leg. Hold for the prescribed time and repeat for other side.

REVERSE CRUNCH

Lie faceup on the floor with your arms at your sides, palms facing down. Keep your feet together. Lift your knees in the air until your hips and knees are at 90 degrees each. Now raise your hips off the floor and crunch them inward—your knees should move toward your chest and your hips and lower back should rise up off the floor (imagine you're emptying a bucket of water that's resting on your pelvis). Pause, then slowly lower your legs until your heels nearly touch the floor.

NOTE: Don't change the bend in your knees from start to finish.

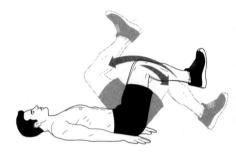

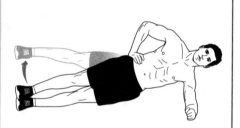

SWISS BALL ROLLOUT

• Sit on your knees in front of a Swiss ball and place your forearms and fists on the ball. Your lower back should be naturally arched and your elbows bent about 90 degrees. While keeping your core braced, slowly roll the ball forward, straightening your arms and extending your body as far as you can without allowing your lower back to "collapse." Pause, then use your abdominal muscles to pull the ball back to your knees.

• Rest 2 minutes.

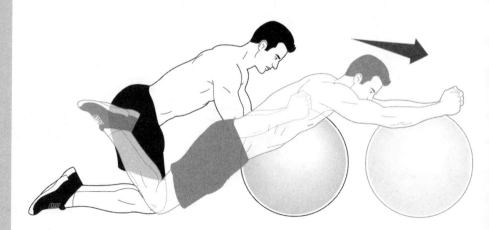

WORKOUT #2: CIRCUIT TWO

CYCLES:
Two to four times through the circuit

ISO-EXPLOSIVE PUSHUP

Assume the pushup position. Bend your elbows and lower your body until your chest nearly touches the floor. Pause 5 seconds in the down position. Then press yourself up so forcefully that your hands leave the floor.

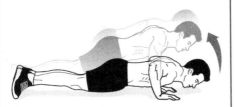

NOTE: This 5-second pause technique eliminates all the elasticity in your muscles, which allows you to activate a maximum number of fast-twitch muscle fibers. These are the fibers with the greatest potential for size and strength gains.

RENEGADE ROW

Select a pair of medium-weight dumbbells and assume a pushup position, feet shoulder-width apart and hands directly beneath your shoulders, gripping the dumbbell handles for support. Minimizing any rolling or tilting in the hips, shift the entire weight of your upper body onto your left hand and pull the dumbbell in your right hand toward your right hip as if performing a single-arm dumbbell row. Lower the dumbbell to the starting position, shift your weight onto your right hand and repeat on the left side. Alternate sides for sets of 10 to 15 repetitions each side.

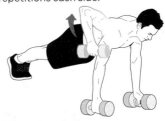

BODY-WEIGHT BULGARIAN SPLIT SQUAT

Stand in a staggered stance, your left foot in front of your right 2 to 3 feet apart. Place just the instep of your back foot on a bench or chair. Pull your shoulders back and brace your core. Lower your body as deeply as you can, keeping your back foot on the bench. Keep your shoulders back and chest up through the movement. Pause, then return to the starting position. Halfway through the prescribed time, switch to the other foot.

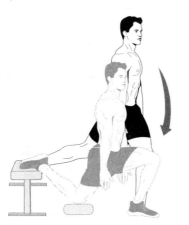

JUMP SQUAT

• Place your fingers on the back of your head and pull your elbows back so that they're in line with your body. Perform a body-weight squat until your thighs are parallel to the floor, then explosively jump as high as you can (imagine you're pushing the floor away from you as you leap). When you land, immediately squat and jump again. Hold dumbbells at your side to make it more challenging.

• Rest 2 minutes.

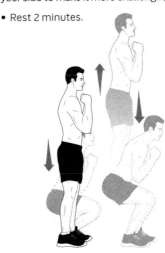

WORKOUT #2: CIRCUIT THREE

CYCLES:
Two to four times through the circuit

MOUNTAIN CLIMBER

Get in pushup position with your arms straight. This is the starting position. Lift your left foot and raise your knee as close to your chest as you can. Touch the ground with your left foot and then return to the starting position and repeat with your right leg. Go as fast as possible.

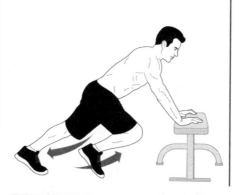

CHINUP

Grab the pullup bar with a shoulder-width, underhand grip. Hang at arm's length. Cross your ankles behind you. You should return to this position—known as a dead hang—each time you lower your body back down. Squeeze your shoulder blades together as you pull your chest to the bar. Once the top of your chest touches the bar, pause, then slowly lower your body back to a dead hang.

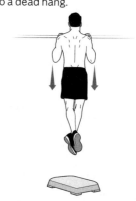

SUICIDES [SHUTTLE RUN]

Sprint five paces, touch the ground, then return to your starting point and touch the ground. Without stopping, now sprint 10 paces, touch the ground, then return to your starting point and touch the ground. Halfway through the prescribed time, start working back down the distance ladder (15 paces, 10 paces, 5 paces, etc.).

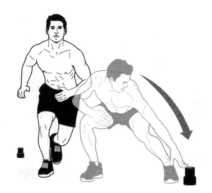

TRX TRICEPS EXTENSION

Face away from the anchor point of a TRX. With one hand in each handle, extend your arms so they're at eye level and walk away from the anchor until you feel tension in the straps. Lean forward so your body is at a 45-degree angle (the shallower the angle, the easier the exercise). Without changing the angle of your upper arms, bend your elbows until your hands are behind your head. Press back to the starting position by driving your hands forward until your arms are straight.

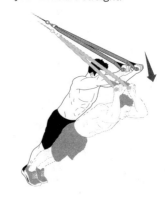

Silver-Level Gut Check and Competition

Now that you've been going full-bore for 6 months, you should return to the three-point fitness check I offered in the previous section and once again test your fitness, keeping the testing parameters as consistent as possible. I imagine you'll surprise yourself once again.

At this point, you also have my permission to dive as fully into competition as you wish. If you've been taking my advice and getting into racing or sports on a regular basis, keep it up. I'd suggest you choose an event that occurs right around the 6-month anniversary of starting your exercise program and sign up for that: maybe a 10-K, which is a healthy-but-doable 6.2 miles, or, if you're into cycling, a half-century bike ride, or, for more adventurous types, an open-water swim of a mile or more. Assuming you've been running, riding, or swimming regularly as your chosen form of cardio, these distances should be a fair challenge for you.

Mud-strewn obstacle courses are getting more and more popular these days, some of which are brutal (the Tough Mudder, for example, based on a special forces obstacle course), and others of which are comparatively mild, assuming you don't mind mud.

Now that you're approaching a pretty decent level of fitness, I suggest you choose your event 2 or 3 months beforehand, and tailor your training to help you peak for it. Better still, enlist some friends to get in on the event as well: Raise some money for a good cause or just have a ball being outside and moving.

"Back to Last":
THE VALUE OF A SUPPORT GROUP

Exercise is medicine, but there are ways to make that medicine even more powerful. For example: Think belonging to a club, a team, or a support group is "just" a social thing? Sometimes it can make all the difference in the world—even, it seems, the difference between life and death.

SEAL Team Physical Training, Inc., is an outdoor, adventure-style, never-the-same twice workout class held in Washington, DC, and northern Virginia. Although not directly affiliated with the military—or intended as a SEAL preparation course—you'd be forgiven for thinking that it was. Like actual SEALs in training, Team PT members sprint, run, climb hills, do bear crawls, crab walks, flutter kicks, back extensions, and pushups by the score. They lift and carry one another across grassy fields, up and over tennis nets and high retaining walls.

There's friendly competition, to be sure, but classes are always a team effort: Finish a run ahead of the group, and you're instructed to go "back to last"— to retrace your steps till you reach the final straggler—and repeat the course from that point on, cheering on your slower teammates. Finish your assigned pushups early and you're told to find a buddy and help him or her work off the rest of theirs. To do any less would be selfish,

narcissistic—contrary to the spirit of the SEALs themselves.

PT founder John McGuire spent 10 years as an actual Navy SEAL, but he's hardly the hard-charging, thick-necked, bull-horn-wielding type you might expect. Compactly built, soft-spoken, quick to smile and offer support, McGuire commands respect in large part by giving it. He eats, sleeps, and breathes the team ethos: We all make it, or none of us do.

Six years ago, this positive-attitude, all-for-one philosophy was put to the ultimate test. Ever the athlete, McGuire was practicing back flips on a trampoline when he took a bad bounce, fell off, and broke his neck. He couldn't move or breathe. Had the paramedics not been speedy, he would have been dead on the scene.

Doctors doubted he'd survive surgery.

When he did, they put his chances of regaining much function at "slim." When they finally discharged him from rehab, they offered him a fancy wheelchair free of charge.

McGuire told them to donate it. He was going to learn to walk again.

So, with the goal of returning to his students firmly in his sights, he crawled, rolled, and wriggled across the floor of his home in Richmond, Virginia, for hours each day, painstakingly relearning first breathing, eating, crawling, and finally, walking—until 3 months later, he was, in fact, coaching again—on his own two feet. No cane. No walker.

Even today, the neurosurgeon who oversaw his recovery says he's a miracle, and wonders how a man pronounced virtually dead on arrival could regain such a high level of functioning in so short a time.

Exercise got him back to this point, as surely as the physical and mental fortitude that McGuire nurtured as an elite soldier helped to carry him through such an agonizing injury and recovery process. But McGuire doesn't talk about that. Instead, he credits his community—the students he teaches, the team leaders he mentors, the prospective SEALS he supports and guides—for helping to get him back on track. Just as he was always there for them, they stepped forward for him, continuing to meet for their brutal workouts every day, carrying on in the tradition he'd taught them. They inundated him with cards, flowers, visits, and constant support. They went "back to last."

Today, with John back at the helm, these students continue to learn from his example. Morning after morning, they see how a person is stronger with a group standing behind him than standing on his own, how working *with* your buddy—as opposed to ignoring, resenting, or trying to trounce him—makes *you* stronger and smarter. "You're not alone in this class," McGuire tells them, "just as you're not alone on this planet. Working together, we can move mountains."

GOLD

THE ADVANCED PROGRAM:
MONTHS 7–9 . . . AND BEYOND

People who have made it to this level in the program—and I sincerely hope that's everyone who started this book—deserve a seriously hearty high-five: You're far, far healthier than you were 6 months ago. You've probably lost a fair amount of fat, gained strength and muscle mass, improved your flexibility, and reset your default mood at a higher and more positive level.

Better still, if I could shrink myself down and drive a mini-submarine through your arteries, the inner walls would appear significantly smoother and cleaner than they did 6 months ago. The blood wouldn't flow as fast and hard since the pressure is down, and also because your heart would be beating less frequently, but much more powerfully, than it did when you started. Altogether, it would be a thoroughly enjoyable ride.

Now it's time to push harder. These advanced workouts will take your fitness and health to another level, giving you a day-to-day energy and performance boost that few people enjoy (because they don't exercise, of course). You've done amazing things so far. Let's finish the job.

The Next Level Is Within Reach

The following exercise routines are incredibly effective, but even at this level, there are a few more things you can do on top of sweating that will boost your results. Now is a good time to talk about them so you can think about adding them before relaunching your program.

- **Commit to Eating Right:** I mentioned this briefly in the Silver section. It's just as important here. You've got to fuel yourself well. If you still have a few eating habits you'd like to improve on, commit to rooting them out as soon, and as thoroughly, as you can. See Part 4 for simple food changes that will yield huge results.

- **Let Enjoyment Be Your Guide:** From here on out, you will start to become more of an expert on what

CHANGE IT UP!

As a triathlete, I may be biased, but there may well be some benefit to the multi-tasking approach that's required when you pursue more than one exercise discipline. As I've said before, the body is highly adaptable: Whatever you ask it to do, it will do its darnedest to do well. Cycle a lot, for example, and the muscles in your hips, thighs, and calves will get bigger and stronger; your heart and lungs become more efficient at supplying oxygen to those muscles; you even start to metabolize your food in ways that can support your hours in the saddle.

Adaptation also requires rest. Your body needs time to build new muscle, connective tissue, capillaries, and neural pathways. If you keep placing the same demands on your body day after day, without letting it rest and recoup, chances are it will eventually break down. Pro athletes have to walk a fine line between training enough so that they stay on top of their game and training so much that they get injured, simply because their livelihood depends on it.

And quite often, rather understandably, the demands of their profession force them to step over that line.

Average weekend warriors make the same mistakes. I see scores of cases of tennis elbow and golfer's knee among average, non-pro Joes and Janes—just regular folks who can't bear to pass up yet another chance to play their favorite sport, no matter the cost.

Fitness teacher and author Frank Forencich recommends taking a seasonal approach to fitness. Some people do this instinctively: swimming in the summer, cross-country skiing in the winter, and so on. Even single-sport athletes do something similar, breaking their training year into an off-season, a preseason, an in-season, and sometimes a postseason, each of which serves specific goals to the athlete. You don't have to be that precise about it, but you should understand that you'll avoid injury, perform better, and enjoy your fitness program more if you switch it up periodically.

your body needs week-to-week and month-to-month than I am. At this level, you'll see that I'm going to offer you even more leeway as far as the activities you do and the time you spend doing each one.

• **Recover, Recover, Recover:** Since your transition from sedentary to seriously athletic has been relatively quick, you may not have noticed that your need for sleep and rest may very well have increased (though your ability to get good sleep may have also improved!), and that your body will now appreciate massage, steam baths, gentle yoga, and other recovery modalities even more than when you started. Go ahead and treat yourself to these things as often as you are able: At least once a month and ideally as often as once a week. You'll notice a big difference in how your body feels.

GOLD
MONTH 1 TRAINING SCHEDULE

During all 3 months of the Gold Level, your weekly workouts will adhere to the following guidelines:

• 2–3 strength-training sessions
• 2–3 cardio sessions, interval or medium-intensity cardio
• For a total of 5 sessions

ALSO:

• 5 dynamic-stretching routines (prior to workouts above)
• 3 foam-rolling routines

• At least one walk of 40 minutes or more
• All the "NEAT" you can handle

Similar to last month, you've got plenty of choices. Since the workouts are getting more specific and intense, I'm going to suggest that you choose either a "cardio track" or a "strength-and-conditioning" track this month, the better to maximize your results. If you like cardio work and are trying to build up to run a solid 10-K, for example, you might arrange your workouts like this:

YOUR GOLD MONTH 1 ROUTINE

MONDAY:	Dynamic stretching, foam rolling, 30-minute long run, fast pace
TUESDAY:	Dynamic stretching, strength training
WEDNESDAY:	Dynamic stretching, foam rolling, interval training (2-minute runs x 4–6, 2 minutes rest)
THURSDAY:	1 hour walk
FRIDAY:	Dynamic stretching, strength training
SATURDAY:	Dynamic stretching, foam rolling, 45-minute run, moderate pace.
SUNDAY:	Easy walk *or* hike, 1 hour

If your focus is on changing your body composition—gaining muscle and losing fat—you'll want to choose the strength-and-conditioning track, which might look like this:

YOUR GOLD MONTH 1 ROUTINE

MONDAY: Dynamic stretching, foam rolling, strength training

TUESDAY: Dynamic stretching, 30-minute run, moderate pace

WEDNESDAY: Dynamic stretching, foam rolling, strength training, *and* short interval training (Tabata stair running)

THURSDAY: 1-hour walk

FRIDAY: Dynamic stretching, foam rolling, strength training

SATURDAY: Dynamic stretching, interval training (cycling)

SUNDAY: Easy walk *or* hike, 1 hour

On Wednesday of the schedule above, you'll see that you're doing both strength-training and interval work during the same workout. That's allowed, but use such "stacked" workouts judiciously, placing them before and after days when you're doing less challenging workouts. Monitor your energy to make sure that it's something you can handle, and if you start to feel overly fatigued or sore on weeks when you double up your workouts in this way, stop doing it.

At this point in your training, you should also become even more attuned to the little signals your body sends about what you're up for on a given day. Are you sore in the morning? How's your energy throughout the day? How are your aches and pains? How's your focus? Even little details like your typing skill one day to the next can provide clues about the state of your nervous system and how well you're recovering from your workouts. When you're tired, back off a bit, but if you're feeling great, go ahead and push harder.

Always, however, complete your full warmup and an exercise or two before making your final evaluation. Many times I've gone into a workout feeling like I wasn't up for it, only to feel incredibly good 5 minutes later.

GOLD
MONTH 1 STRENGTH-TRAINING OVERVIEW

This month you're going to venture into the gym for your strength-training workouts. Basic barbell weight training and using challenging loads are skills that every exerciser should have. As good as body-weight training can be, there's something about lifting steadily heavier weights week to week and getting steadily more skilled at the basic exercises that is extremely satisfying, and makes the body respond like no other form of exercise. It's unquestionably the best way to build muscle mass, and if you commit to it and work hard, the physical changes can be substantial, and can happen quickly.

However: No one—least of all women—should worry about getting "too big" from strength training, any more than they should worry about getting "too fast" from running or "too lean" from dieting. The physical changes that occur from lifting heavy weights can be significant, but they don't happen overnight, and they don't happen by accident, either. On the program that follows, I suspect that if anything you'll be very pleased with the results you get and if anything will want more of them.

Among the many other advan-tages of lifting heavy is the fact that you can so easily control the difficulty of the exercise. If it's too hard, lift a little less weight. Too easy, lift a little more. That's a huge advantage, particularly if ever you find yourself having to rehab after an injury or illness. There's an entry point for everyone.

Starting on the next page, you will find your two strength-training workouts for the month. Perform them alternately, on nonconsecutive days, doing either two or three sessions each week, depending on whether you've chosen the strength track or the cardio track this month. On each of the "paired" exercises, alternate a set of the first exercise with a set of the second until you've completed 3 sets of each exercise. On each move, choose a weight that challenges you to complete all the reps listed with good form, and strive to increase the weight you lift by a small amount every week.

WORKOUT #1

CORE CIRCUIT: Perform each exercise for a total of 50 seconds, getting as many good-form reps as you can, before resting 10 seconds and moving on to the next exercise. Go twice through this core circuit, doing just one side on Turkish get-ups on each time through.

SWISS BALL ROLLOUT

Sit on your knees in front of a Swiss ball and place your forearms and fists on the ball. Your lower back should be naturally arched and your elbows bent about 90 degrees. While keeping your core braced, slowly roll the ball forward, straightening your arms and extending your body as far as you can without allowing your lower back to "collapse." Pause, then use your abdominal muscles to pull the ball back to your knees.

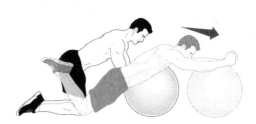

LYING HANDS-TO-FEET BALL PASS

Lie on your back, holding a small- to medium-size Swiss ball in your hands directly over your head. Forcefully bracing your core and pressing your lower back toward the floor, lift your legs until they are pointed directly toward the ceiling. With your head relaxed on the floor, transfer the ball from your hands to your legs, gripping it with your lower legs and feet. Keeping your thighs pointed straight up, bend your knees and lower the ball until it is a couple of inches from the floor. As you lower your legs, simultaneously reach and stretch your arms toward the floor over your head, keeping them parallel. With your lower back pressed toward the floor, raise your arms and legs until they are above your torso again, and transfer the ball from your legs to your hands. Lower your hands and feet toward the floor again, this time holding the ball with your hands. Bring the arms and legs back to the starting position and transfer the ball back to your feet. Count 1 rep each time you transfer the ball.

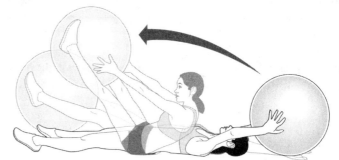

TURKISH GET-UP (ONE SIDE EACH TIME THROUGH THE CYCLE)

Lie faceup with your legs straight. Hold a dumbbell in your left hand with your arm straight above you. Don't take your eyes off the dumbbell at any time. Roll onto your right side and prop yourself up on your right elbow. Place your left foot flat on the floor, then push yourself into a position with your right knee down and your left foot still flat on the floor. Simply stand up, while keeping your arm straight and the dumbbell above you at all times. Once standing, reverse the movement to return to the starting position.

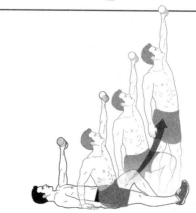

PAIR A (alternate sets of these exercises until you perform 3 sets of each, then move to Pair B):

1A. DEADLIFT (6–8 REPS)

Load a barbell and roll it against your shins. Bend at your hips and knees and grab the bar with an overhand grip, your hands just beyond shoulder width. Without allowing your lower back to round, pull your torso back and up, thrust your hips forward, and stand up with the barbell. Squeeze your glutes as you perform the movement. Lower the bar to the floor, keeping it as close to your body as possible.

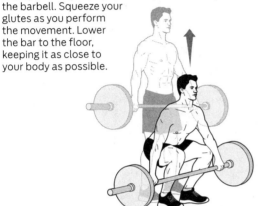

2A. INCLINE DUMBBELL BENCH PRESS (6–8 REPS)

Set an adjustable bench to its lowest incline, about 15 to 30 degrees. Lie faceup on the bench and hold the dumbbells above your shoulders, with your arms straight. Bring the dumbbells down to the sides of your upper chest. Pause, then press the weights back up to the starting position.

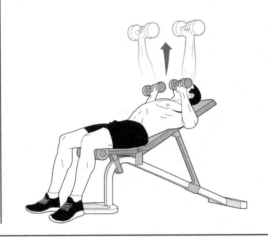

PAIR B (alternate sets of these exercises until you perform 3 sets of each):

1B. BODY-WEIGHT BULGARIAN SPLIT SQUAT (6–8 REPS PER LEG)

Stand in a staggered stance, your left foot in front of your right 2 to 3 feet apart. Place just the instep of your back foot on a bench or chair. Pull your shoulders back and brace your core. Lower your body as deeply as you can, keeping your back foot on the bench. Keep your shoulders back and chest up through the movement. Pause, then return to the starting position. Halfway through the prescribed time, switch to the other foot.

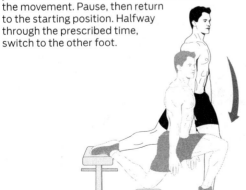

2B. SEATED CABLE ROW (6–8 REPS)

Attach a straight bar to a cable station and sit in front of it with your feet braced. Grab the bar with an over-hand grip that's just beyond shoulder width. Sit up straight and push your chest out and pull your shoulders down and back. Without moving your torso, pull the bar to your upper abs. Pause, then slowly return to the starting position.

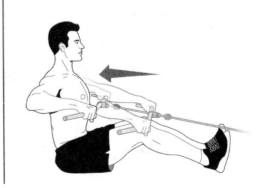

WORKOUT #2

CORE CIRCUIT:

Perform each exercise for a total of 50 seconds, getting as many good-form reps as you can before resting 10 seconds and moving on to the next exercise. Go twice through this core circuit, doing just one side on the side plank each time through.

BARBELL ROLLOUT

Load a barbell with 10-pound plates and affix collars. Kneel on the floor and grab the bar with an overhand, shoulder-width grip. Your shoulders should start over the barbell. Slowly roll the bar forward, extending your body as far as you can without allowing your hips to sag (brace your core and squeeze your glutes to help you keep form). Use your abdominal muscles to pull the bar back to the starting position.

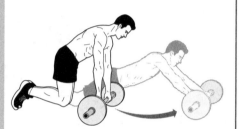

ELBOW-TO-KNEE CRUNCH

Lie faceup with your hips and knees bent 90 degrees so that your lower legs are parallel to the floor. Place your fingers on the sides of your head. Lift your shoulders off the floor as if doing a crunch. Twist your upper body to the left while bringing up your left knee to touch your right elbow. Simultaneously straighten your right leg. Return to the starting position and repeat to the other side.

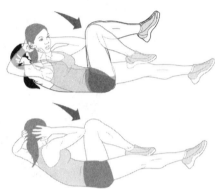

SIDE PLANK WITH TOP LEG RAISE

(ONE SIDE EACH TIME THROUGH THE CYCLE)

Lie on your side and use your forearm to support your body. One ankle should be on top of the other. Raise your hips until your body forms a straight line from shoulder to ankles. Now lift your top leg until it's a foot to 18 inches above the bottom leg. Hold for the prescribed time and repeat for the other side.

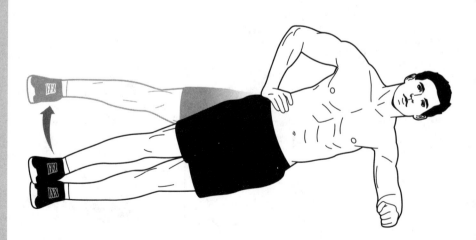

PAIR A (alternate sets of these exercises until you perform 3 sets of each, then move to Pair B):

1A. GOBLET SQUAT (8–10 REPS)

Hold a dumbbell vertically next to your chest with both hands gripping the dumbbell head (you can also grip a kettlebell). Brace your core and lower your body as far as you can by pushing your hips back and bending your knees. Pause, then slowly push yourself back to the starting position.

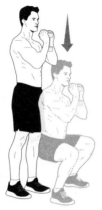

2A. PULLUP

(ASSISTED IF NECESSARY, 8–10 REPS)

Grab the pullup bar with a shoulder-width, overhand grip. Hang at arm's length. Cross your ankles behind you. You should return to this position—known as a dead hang—each time you lower your body back down. Squeeze your shoulder blades together as you pull your chest to the bar. Once the top of your chest touches the bar, pause, then slowly lower your body back to a dead hang.

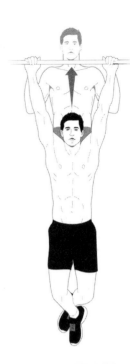

PAIR B (alternate sets of these exercises until you perform 3 sets of each):

1B. ALTERNATING STEP-UP WITH DUMBBELLS (10–12 REPS PER FOOT)

Hold a dumbbell in each hand at arm's length next to your sides. Stand in front of a bench or step and place your right foot firmly on the step. Press your heel into the step and push your body up until your right leg is straight. Pause for a second, then lower your body back down until your left foot touches the floor. Switch feet, then repeat.

2B. BARBELL SHOULDER PRESS

(10–12 REPS)

Grab a barbell with an overhand grip that's just beyond shoulder width and hold it at shoulder level in front of your body. Stand with your feet shoulder-width apart, knees slightly bent. Brace your core. Push the barbell straight overhead, leaning your head back slightly but keeping your torso upright. Pause, then slowly lower your body back to the starting position.

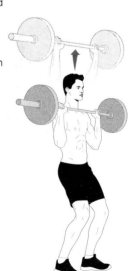

GOLD
MONTH 1
CARDIO TRAINING

If you've chosen the cardio track this month, the main new element will be longer moderate-intensity sessions. In prior months, those workouts have lasted no more than about 30 minutes. This month, you can extend that up to 45 minutes (or even an hour, if you feel strong). As always, monitor your energy to make sure you're recovering optimally between sessions.

If you've chosen the strength-and-conditioning track, this month I suggest you dial back on moderate cardio and emphasize easy walks and interval training instead. The reason is that I want you to experience the *maximum* benefit you can get from higher-intensity training, and the best way to do that is by cutting back a little on the jogging and longer, slower distance work.

GOLD
MONTH 2
TRAINING SCHEDULE

This month, if you stick with a cardio track you'll do three tough cardio workouts and just two strength workouts per week. If you go with a strength-and-conditioning track, you'll do three strength workouts and just two cardio workouts. Here's what it will look like:

- 2–3 strength-training sessions
- 2–3 cardio sessions, interval or medium-intensity cardio
- For a total of 5 sessions

ALSO:

- 5 dynamic-stretching routines (prior to workouts above)
- 3 foam-rolling routines
- At least one walk of 40 minutes or more
- All the "NEAT" you can handle

The cardio track might look like this:

YOUR GOLD MONTH 2 ROUTINE	
MONDAY:	Dynamic stretching, foam rolling, 30-minute run, fast pace
TUESDAY:	Dynamic stretching, strength training
WEDNESDAY:	Dynamic stretching, foam rolling, interval training (2-minute runs x 4–6, 2 minutes rest)
THURSDAY:	1-hour walk
FRIDAY:	Dynamic stretching, strength training
SATURDAY:	Dynamic stretching, foam rolling, 45-minute run, moderate pace
SUNDAY:	Easy walk *or* hike, 1 hour

The strength-and-conditioning track might look like this:

YOUR GOLD MONTH 2 ROUTINE

MONDAY: Dynamic stretching, foam rolling, strength training

TUESDAY: Dynamic stretching, 30-minute run, moderate pace

WEDNESDAY: Dynamic stretching, foam rolling, strength training *and* short interval training (Tabata stair running)

THURSDAY: 1-hour walk

FRIDAY: Dynamic stretching, foam rolling, strength training

SATURDAY: Dynamic stretching, interval training (cycling)

SUNDAY: Easy walk *or* hike, 1 hour

Your strength workouts will be the heaviest and toughest yet, so take a week of workouts to learn the new movements and find your groove before you really start to challenge yourself with big weights. As in previous months, there are two strength workouts this month, Workout A and Workout B, which you should perform alternately each time you do a strength-training workout. If you do two strength-training workouts a week, that means you'll always do Workout A on your first strength-training day of the week and Workout B on your second day. If you do three a week, you'll wind up doing two Workout A's and one Workout B one week, and two B's and one A the next.

With cardio, the goal this month should be increasing your speed. You're already fit in a general sense—so now it's time to think about *performance*. How fit can you get?

At the beginning of this month, I want you to measure your cardio fitness. Here's how:

- Choose a cardio routine you do regularly that usually takes you about a half hour.

- Warm up thoroughly for 10 to 15 minutes.

- Perform the routine at a racing pace: your top speed you think you can maintain for the entire route. Try to finish strong.

- As you did on previous tests, make a note of your finish time.

As you've done in previous months with other fitness tests, you'll check yourself again on the same route at the end of this month. Even if you don't run races regularly, knowing you've got a goal to beat 4 weeks from now will help you push your cardio workouts a little harder throughout the month.

All right—let's get sweaty!

WORKOUT #1

CORE CIRCUIT:
Perform each exercise for a total of 50 seconds, getting as many good-form reps as you can, before resting for 10 seconds and moving on to the next exercise. Go twice through this core circuit, doing just one side on the plank each time through.

SIDE PLANK WITH TOP LEG RAISE
(ONE SIDE EACH TIME THROUGH THE CYCLE)
Lie on your side and use your forearm to support your body. One ankle should be on top of the other. Raise your hips until your body forms a straight line from shoulder to ankles. Now lift your top leg until it's a foot to 18 inches above the bottom leg.

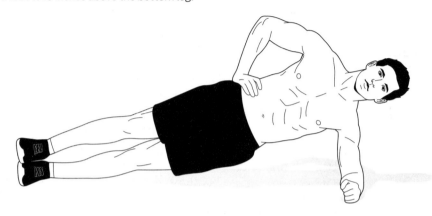

SWISS BALL TOE TOUCHDOWN

Assume a pushup position with the tops of your feet elevated on a medium-size Swiss ball. Make sure your body forms a straight line: your head and neck in line with your spine, and your shoulders over your hands.

Keeping the upper body as motionless as possible and your knees straight, lift your left leg a few inches off the Swiss ball. Extend your left leg to the left of the ball and lower it slowly, tapping the floor with your toes at the bottom of the movement. Slowly lift your left leg back up to rest on top of the ball. Repeat the movement with your right leg, and alternate sides for a total of up to 15 reps on each side. Perform 2 to 3 sets.

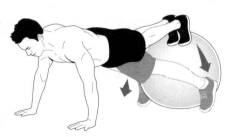

V-UP
Lie faceup on the floor with your legs straight and your arms straight above the top of your head, in line with your body. In one movement, simultaneously lift your torso and legs as if you're trying to touch your toes. Keep your head in line with your body; don't crane your neck. Your legs should be straight and your torso and legs should form a V. Lower your body back to the starting position.

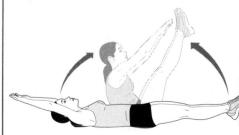

PAIR A (alternate sets of these exercises until you perform 4 sets of each, then move to Pair B):

1A. DEADLIFT (5 REPS)

Load a barbell and roll it against your shins. Bend at your hips and knees and grab the bar with an overhand grip, your hands just beyond shoulder width. Without allowing your lower back to round, pull your torso back and up, thrust your hips forward, and stand up with the barbell. Squeeze your glutes as you perform the movement. Lower the bar to the floor, keeping it as close to your body as possible.

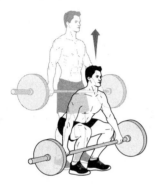

2A. BENCH PRESS (5 REPS)

Grasp a barbell with an overhand grip that's just wider than shoulder width and hold it above your sternum with arms completely straight. Lower the bar straight down, pause, then press the bar in a straight line back up to the starting position. Keep your elbows tucked in so that your upper arms form a 45-degree angle with your body in the down position. This reduces stress on your shoulder joints.

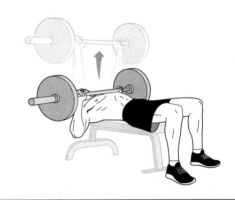

PAIR B (alternate sets of these exercises until you perform 3 sets of each):

1B. OVERHEAD DUMBBELL SQUAT
(10–12 REPS)

Hold a pair of dumbbells over your head at shoulder width. Set your feet shoulder-width apart. Brace your core and lower your body by pushing your hips back and bending your knees until your thighs are parallel to the floor (or lower). Don't allow the dumbbells to move forward as you lower your body.

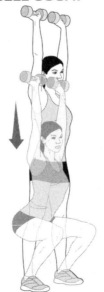

2B. SEATED CABLE ROW
(10–12 REPS)

Attach a straight bar to a cable station and sit in front of it with your feet braced. Grab the bar with an overhand grip that's just beyond shoulder width. Sit up straight and push your chest out and pull your shoulders down and back. Without moving your torso, pull the bar to your upper abs. Pause, then slowly return to the starting position.

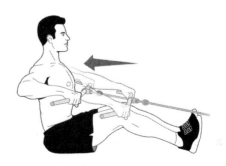

WORKOUT #2

CORE CIRCUIT:

Perform each exercise for a total of 50 seconds, getting as many good-form reps as you can, before resting for 10 seconds and moving on to the next exercise. Go twice through this core circuit, doing just one side on the plank each time through.

WIDE-STANCE PLANK WITH OPPOSITE ARM AND LEG LIFT

• Start to get in the pushup position, but bend your elbows and rest your weight on your forearms instead of on your hands. Your body should form a straight line from your shoulders to your ankles. Move your feet out wider than your shoulders.

• Brace your core by contracting your abs as if you're about to be punched in the gut. Now raise your left foot and right arm off the floor and hold.

SWISS-BALL TOE TOUCHDOWN

Assume a pushup position with the tops of your feet elevated on a medium-size Swiss ball. Make sure your body forms a straight line: your head and neck in line with your spine, and your shoulders over your hands.

Keeping the upper body as motionless as possible and your knees straight, lift your left leg a few inches off the Swiss ball. Extend your left leg to the left of the ball and lower it slowly, tapping the floor with your toes at the bottom of the movement. Slowly lift your left leg back up to rest on top of the ball. Repeat the movement with your right leg, and alternate sides for a total of up to 15 reps on each side. Perform 2 to 3 sets.

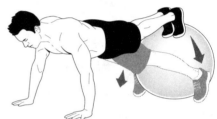

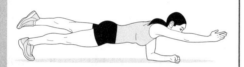

V-UP

Lie faceup on the floor with your legs straight and your arms straight above the top of your head, in line with your body. In one movement, simultaneously lift your torso and legs as if you're trying to touch your toes. Keep your head in line with your body; don't crane your neck. Your legs should be straight and your torso and legs should form a V. Lower your body back to the starting position.

PAIR A (alternate sets of these exercises until you perform *4 sets* of each, then move to Pair B):

1A. OVERHEAD BARBELL LUNGE

(10 REPS PER LEG)
Hold a barbell directly over your shoulders with your arms completely straight. Step forward with your left leg into a lunge. Don't allow the weight to carry you forward. Instead, think about dropping your hips straight down as you step forward.

NOTE: If you have the room to move, do these as walking lunges.

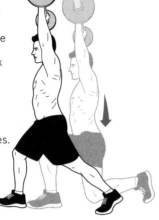

2A. PULLUP

(5 REPS)
Grab the pullup bar with a shoulder-width, overhand grip. Hang at arm's length. Cross your ankles behind you. You should return to this position—known as a dead hang—each time you lower your body back down. Squeeze your shoulder blades together as you pull your chest to the bar. Once the top of your chest touches the bar, pause, then slowly lower your body back to a dead hang.

NOTE: To make this more challenging, vary the width and orientation of your grip on each set.

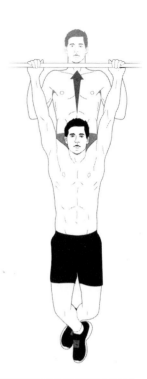

PAIR B (alternate sets of these exercises until you perform *3 sets* of each):

1B. SINGLE-LEG DEADLIFT

(8 REPS PER LEG)
Set a pair of dumbbells on the floor in front of you. Bend at the hips and knees and grab the dumbbells with an overhand grip. Without allowing your lower back to round, stand up with the dumbbells. Now lift your right foot and balance on your left. Bend at your hips and lower your torso until it's almost parallel to the floor. As you bend, your right leg should be straight out behind you. Pause, then raise your torso back to the starting position. Halfway through the prescribed time, switch legs.

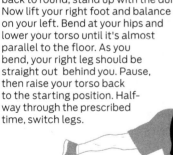

2B. DUMBBELL SHOULDER PRESS

(5 REPS)
Stand holding a pair of dumbbells just outside your shoulders, with your arms bent and palms facing each other. Set your feet shoulder-width apart and slightly bend your knees. Press the weights upward until your arms are completely straight. Slowly lower the dumbbells back to the starting position. Keep your core braced throughout the movement.

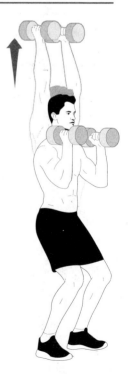

MONTH 3 TRAINING SCHEDULE

You're now the better part of a year into your training, and I imagine you look and feel like a whole new person. I'm going to leave you with one more month of workouts, this time returning to the "hybrid" system you've done in the past. Now that you've spent 2 months building up your strength and power, these body-weight workouts will feel very different: Pushups and squats and pullups will be easier. At the same time, your cardiovascular system, pumped up by all the regular cardio, will be able to power you through the workouts with new vigor.

By now, the format should be familiar:

- 2–3 strength-training sessions

- 2–3 cardio sessions, interval or medium-intensity cardio

- For a total of 5 *sessions*

CAN'T I JUST DO EVERYTHING?

Picture two world-class athletes: one an Olympic weight lifter, the other a marathon runner. Both are, in their own way, extremely healthy and fit, capable of astonishing feats of athleticism. But if you asked these two athletes to swap events, chances are they'd both flame out: The weight lifter might start out strong in the footrace, but would quickly fade as more enduring runners sped by. The marathoner wouldn't have the strength or power to lift a respectable weight.

To an extent, fitness is fitness. A sedentary man or woman who starts a fitness program will get stronger, faster, more flexible, *and* more enduring: It's the rising fitness tide that raises all ships.

But once you reach a certain threshold, further development of some of these fitness qualities starts to inhibit the development of others. Long-distance runners, for instance, need a high level of *capillary density* in their legs so that oxygen can be delivered to the muscles with maximum efficiency. Weight lifters, on the other hand, benefit from stronger, larger muscles, whose capillaries are necessarily less densely packed than the runner's. The two activities place unique demands on the body that, to some degree, work against one another, a phenomenon known as the *interference effect*.

Does that mean you necessarily have to choose one activity or another? No. Weight lifters *do* benefit from some cardio work, just as long-distance runners benefit from some strength and power work.

If you find yourself itching to commit more fully to a particular sport or activity, go for it. But even the specialists know it's a mistake to dial any aspect of your fitness program down to absolutely zero.

ALSO:

- 5 dynamic-stretching routines (prior to workouts above)

- 3 foam-rolling routines

- At least one walk of 40 minutes or more

- All the "NEAT" you can handle

The cardio track might look like this:

YOUR GOLD MONTH 3 ROUTINE

MONDAY:	Dynamic stretching, foam rolling, 30-minute run, fast pace
TUESDAY:	Dynamic stretching, strength training
WEDNESDAY:	Dynamic stretching, foam rolling, interval training (2-minute runs x 4–6, 2 minutes rest)
THURSDAY:	1-hour walk
FRIDAY:	Dynamic stretching, strength training
SATURDAY:	Dynamic stretching, foam rolling, 45-minute run, moderate pace
SUNDAY:	Easy walk or hike, 1 hour

The strength-and-conditioning track might look like this:

YOUR GOLD MONTH 3 ROUTINE

MONDAY:	Dynamic stretching, foam rolling, strength training
TUESDAY:	Dynamic stretching, 30-minute run, moderate pace
WEDNESDAY:	Dynamic stretching, foam rolling, strength training *and* short interval training (Tabata stair running)
THURSDAY:	1-hour walk
FRIDAY:	Dynamic stretching, foam rolling, strength training
SATURDAY:	Dynamic stretching, interval training (cycling)
SUNDAY:	Easy walk or hike, 1 hour

GOLD
MONTH 3 STRENGTH TRAINING

Here are your strength-training workouts for the month. Perform each exercise for 50 seconds; rest for 10, and move on to the next. Repeat each group of exercises for the indicated number of cycles.

YOUR FINAL EXAM: DO SOMETHING

Since you're going to be finishing the program at the end of this month, I'm going to actually *require* that you find yourself a fitness challenge—ideally something that you do with others, in an organized setting, and sign up. It can be a road race, a mountain bike race, a long mountain climb, or even a serious swim. Whatever it is, do it. Whether you just started at the gold level, or whether you've been at this for 9 months, it's important that you find a way to mark this occasion in some significant way. It's your version of the "black belt" test: a public declaration of your ongoing dedication to health and fitness.

WORKOUT #1

Perform the maximum reps in 50 seconds, rest 10 seconds, then move to the next exercise. Perform each circuit three times.

1A. BODY-WEIGHT SQUAT

Place your fingers on the back of your head and pull your elbows back so that they're in line with your body. Perform a body-weight squat until your thighs are parallel to the floor, then rise back to the starting position.

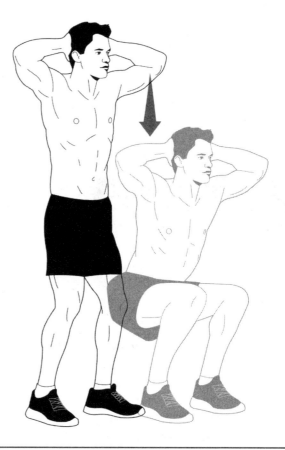

1B. PUSHUP

Get into pushup position gripping hexagonal dumbbells in your hands as a base, if you want to make it more interesting. Keeping your body straight from your head to your ankles, lower your body until your chest nearly touches the floor. Pause at the bottom and then push yourself back to the starting position as quickly as possible.

1C. TREADMILL/ JUMP ROPE/ STATIONARY BIKE, 50 SECONDS

Rest 2 minutes.

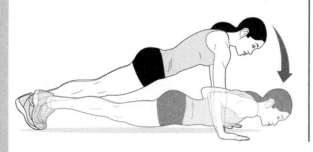

2A. ELBOW-TO-KNEE CRUNCH

Lie faceup with your hips and knees bent 90 degrees so that your lower legs are parallel to the floor. Place your fingers on the sides of your head. Lift your shoulders off the floor as if doing a crunch. Twist your upper body to the right while bringing up your right knee to touch your left elbow. Simultaneously straighten your left leg. Return to the starting position and repeat to the other side.

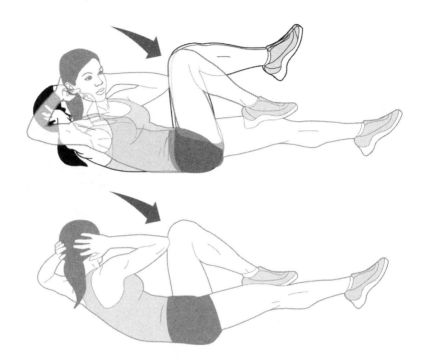

2B. MOUNTAIN CLIMBER

Get in pushup position with your arms straight. This is the starting position. Lift your left foot and raise your knee as close to your chest as you can. Touch the ground with your left foot and then return to the starting position and repeat with your right leg. Go as fast as possible.

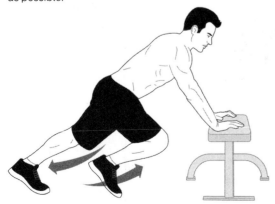

2C. PLANK

• Get into pushup position but bend your elbows and rest your weight on your forearms. Your body should form a straight line from your shoulders to your ankles. Brace your core and hold.

• Rest 2 minutes.

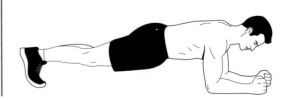

WORKOUT #1—*Continued*

3A. BODY-WEIGHT BULGARIAN SPLIT SQUAT

Stand in a staggered stance, your left foot in front of your right 2 to 3 feet apart. Place just the instep of your back foot on a bench or chair. Pull your shoulders back and brace your core. Lower your body as deeply as you can, keeping your back foot on the bench. Keep your shoulders back and chest up through the movement. Pause, then return to the starting position. Halfway through the prescribed time, switch to the other foot.

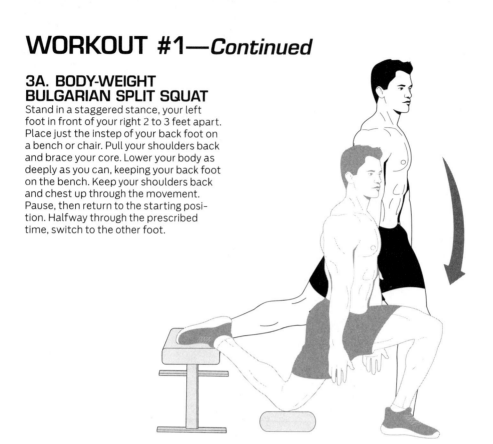

3B. TRX ROW

Hold a TRX handle in each hand and back away until you feel tension in the straps. Your body should form a 45- to 60-degree angle to the floor (the deeper the angle, the harder the exercise), and your arms should be parallel to the floor, palms down. Pull your body toward the anchor point by bringing the handles to the sides of your chest as you rotate your palms inward. Your elbows should be at 45 degrees. Pause and return to the starting position.

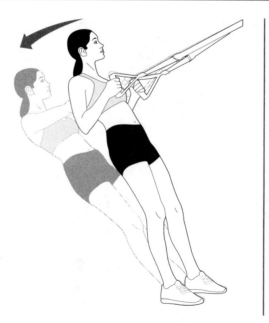

3C. TREADMILL/ JUMP ROPE/ STATIONARY BIKE SPRINT, 50 SECONDS

WORKOUT #2

Perform the maximum reps in 50 seconds, rest 10 seconds, then move to the next exercise. Perform each circuit 3 times

1A. SINGLE-ARM DUMBBELL/ KETTLEBELL SWING

Hold a dumbbell (or kettlebell) at arm's length in front of your waist. Without rounding your lower back, bend at your hips and knees and swing the dumbbell between your legs. Keeping your arm straight, thrust your hips forward and swing the dumbbell to shoulder level as you rise to a standing position. Swing the weight back and forth. Halfway through your time, switch arms.

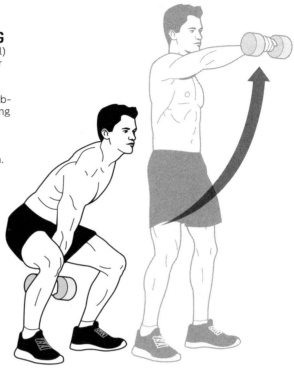

1B. PUSHUP

Get into pushup position with your hands shoulder-width apart. Keeping your body straight from your head to your ankles, lower your body until your chest nearly touches the floor. Pause at the bottom and then push yourself back to the starting position as quickly as possible.

1C. TREADMILL/ JUMP ROPE/ STEP MILL SPRINT, 50 SECONDS

Rest 2 minutes.

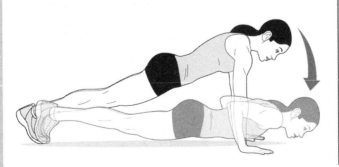

WORKOUT #2—*Continued*

2A. ROLLING SIDE PLANK

Start by performing a side plank with your right side down. Hold for 1 or 2 seconds, then roll your body over—into a traditional pushup position—and hold for 1 or 2 seconds. Next, roll all the way up onto your left elbow so that you're performing a side plank facing the opposite direction. Hold for another second or two. That's 1 repetition. Make sure to move your whole body as a single unit each time you roll.

2B. CORE STABILIZATION

• Sit on the floor with your knees bent. Hold a weight plate straight out in front of your chest. Your feet should be flat on the floor. Lean back so your torso is at a 45-degree angle to the floor, and brace your core.

• Without moving your torso (your belly button should point straight ahead at all times), rotate your arms to the left as far as you can. Pause for 3 seconds. Rotate your arms to the right as far as you can. Pause again, then continue to alternate back and forth.

NOTE: If you don't have a weight plate, you can substitute a light dumbbell, a basketball, a rock, or if you have no object (or need the exercise to be easier), simply clasp your hands together in front of you.

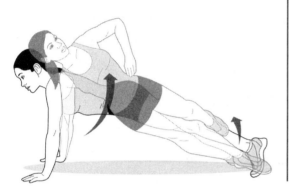

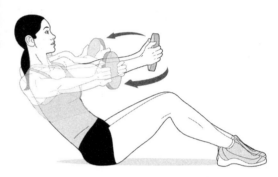

2C. SWISS BALL PIKE

• Assume the pushup position with your arms completely straight and your hands slightly wider than your shoulders. Rest your shins on a Swiss ball. Your body should form a straight line from your head to your ankles. Without bending your knees, roll the Swiss ball toward your body by raising your hips as high as you can. Don't round your lower back. Pause, then return the ball to the starting position by lowering your hips and rolling the ball backward.

• Rest 2 minutes.

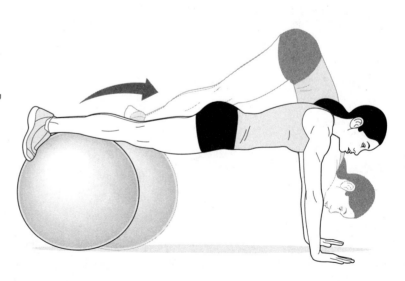

3A. SPLIT JUMP

Stand in a staggered stance, your left foot in front of your right. Lower your body as far as you can. Quickly switch directions and jump with enough force to propel both feet off the floor. While in the air, scissor-kick your legs so you land with the opposite leg forward. Repeat, alternating back and forth with each repetition.

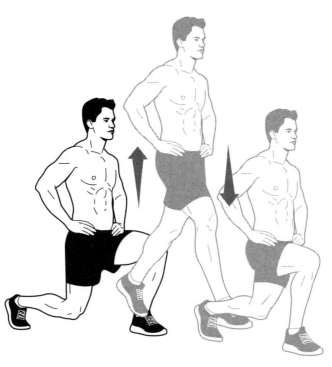

3B. PULLUP

Grab the pullup bar with a shoulder-width, overhand grip. Hang at arm's length. Cross your ankles behind you. You should return to this position—known as a dead hang—each time you lower your body back down. Squeeze your shoulder blades together as you pull your chest to the bar. Once the top of your chest touches the bar, pause, then slowly lower your body back to a dead hang.

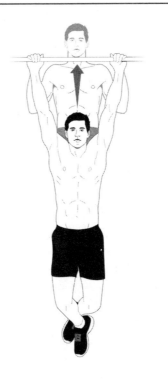

3C. TREADMILL/ JUMP ROPE/ STATIONARY BIKE SPRINT, 50 SECONDS

The By-Laws of Strength Training

So far in this program, I've spelled everything out explicitly: which exercises to do, what order, how many reps, and so on. Now that you're at the end of the Gold Level—and about to strike off on your own—I want to "teach you to fish," to train with a goal in mind and an eye toward improvement. To do that, you've got to know your way around the gym. Use these tips as your GPS.

1. Stick with Compound Moves:

Go into the average gym and you'll encounter dozens of different machines and hundreds of different exercise variations. How do you know which ones to do? Here's a simple rule: If you're moving two or more joints when you do the move, it's a keeper. One joint? Optional at best.

Picture two different exercises that involve your arms. The first move is a dumbbell curl: You hold the weight at arm's length by your side and curl it up to shoulder height, reverse the move and repeat. For all intents and purposes, all the movement is happening around the elbow joint.

Now picture a chinup: Your elbow joint moves in a similar way. But now you're moving at the shoulder joint, too. If you look carefully, your spine is also doing a little undulation movement that your core muscles have to control. Heck, even your legs have to get in on the action a little bit.

With the chinup, in other words, you're getting all the biceps-building benefit of the barbell curl—but you're working a whole lot of other muscle groups at the same time as well. So working your muscles in groups in this way is simply more time-efficient than working all the 600 of them in isolation.

It also works better. The body seems to understand compound movements better than it does isolation exercises. If you push or pull something heavy using lots of different muscle groups at once, it seems to flip an evolutionary switch that makes muscles grow and get stronger. Not so with isolation moves.

2. Balance Your Exercises:

Any strength-training exercise worth its salt will break down into one of the following categories:

- Any core exercise.

- Any exercise where you *squat* downward with a weight at shoulder height or above, including front squats, overhead squats, and back squats.

- Any exercise where you pull, or *deadlift* a weight from the ground, including straight-leg, sumo, and standard versions.

- Any exercise where you *pull* a load toward you. Rows and chinups are great examples.

- Any exercise that you perform with a *split stance* or *on one leg,* including all lunges, step-ups, and single-leg squats.

- Any exercise where you *push* a load away from you, such as a bench press.

There are hybrid moves: A pushup, for example, is a core move and a pushing move. A split squat to overhead press is a single-leg move and a press. But these are the basic categories. When in doubt, do a workout that includes a balance of exercises from these six categories.

Men and women favor different types of exercises: Guys like to bench press to build their pecs; women tend to emphasize their thighs and glutes. There's nothing wrong with those exercises, as long as you don't focus on them to the exclusion of other important moves.

3. Use Free Weights, Not Machines:

Machines can be great for novices or injured people. But for everyone else, they're not a great use of time. Why? Again, it comes down to a question of isolating muscle groups versus using many muscles at once. When you sit in a seat and push a loaded platform with your legs, as on a leg press machine, there's no need for you to balance or stabilize that weight. If you squat while holding two dumbbells at shoulder height, on the other hand, your core and back musculature have to work hard to protect your spine and keep you upright; your ankles, hips, and knees now have to work to balance you as well as to power the weight up. This makes the exercise more *functional*—applicable to sport, recreation, and everyday life. The only application I can think of for the leg press machine is if you happen get pinned under something heavy with

your legs conveniently braced against it, and your need to launch it off you with your legs. Can't think of a time that's ever happened to me, but if it comes up a lot in your line of work, go ahead and leg press all you want.

4. Variety:

The number one complaint about strength training? It's boring. The way most people do it—repeating the same program, with the same 10 exercises, for months at a time, well, I fully agree! A strength-training program needs to grow and change along with you, so it never gets too easy and it never gets dull.

If you're stumped for what to do in the gym, and want to shake things up, do *any* core move, any squat *or* a deadlift, any pulling move, any single-leg move, and any pushing move, *in that order*. Do about 3 sets of 8 to 10 reps on each move, using challenging weights. You'll be prioritizing well, and you'll be hitting every muscle in relatively short order.

5. Progression:

The old-fashioned strength-and-conditioning guys used to call strength exercise "progressive resistance training." At some point, people got tired of wasting the ink and just dropped the word "progression."

In truth, all exercise *should* be progressive: You should be trying to get stronger, faster, more flexible, more enduring, pretty much all the time, for your whole life. But it rarely works out that way: Instead, we tend to get comfortable doing a certain number of reps with a certain amount of weight, and we settle for "good enough." Then, over time, the "good enough" bar tends to backslide over time, and our fitness starts to fade.

The solution? Keep it progressive. That doesn't always mean just throwing more weight on a bar. It can mean doing more reps, more sets, or even—and this isn't used as much—a tougher version of the same exercise. Body-weight squats are a great move, but at some point, they become manageable. Doing them on one leg can solve that little problem but quick.

6. Rest: When all else fails in a strength-training program—when you're sore, and not getting stronger, and would rather have a root canal than hit the weights again—take a few days off. Even up to a week. I don't talk about this much in previous levels, because it can sound like an excuse to slack off. But your body can only take so much stress before it breaks down. If you're an exercise fiend like me, you may want to climb the walls during those days off. But when you come back, trust me, you'll come back stronger.

Beyond the Finish Line: Where to Go from Here?

Fitness pros like to point out the difference between training and activity: "Training" is goal-driven, part of an overall plan to get you healthier,

stronger, faster, leaner. Regular training means you're at least somewhat aware of what you did yesterday, last month, and last year, and have an eye focused on what you want to accomplish tomorrow, *next* month, and *next* year. "Activity" is free-form: You go for a walk, play a game of tennis, go for a hike for enjoyment, but not necessarily with a clear goal in mind. You're doing it because it's fun and feels good. All NEAT, by definition, falls under this heading: It's activity, as opposed to training.

Both training and activity have their place, even in a serious exercise program. And if you're doing either one, you're aces in my book. But as a Gold-Level exerciser preparing to move on in the world, you'll want to spend a larger portion of your exercise time on "training."

Why? After your first few months as a regular exerciser, regular old activity won't effect much visible change in your health, performance, or appearance. In order to keep progressing, then, you've got to raise the bar on yourself, again and again. And to do that, you've got to *train:* to find ways to get better *systematically.*

At this point in your exercise program, you probably have a pretty good grasp of what attributes of fitness are your strong points, and which are your weaker ones. Maybe long cardio workouts have always felt good to you (as they always have to me), but intervals and strength training haven't. Or maybe you love speed training but hate plodding slowly along for mile after mile.

If you're after across-the-board, general fitness, you'll want to include at least some strength work and some cardio work as you continue along the path to greater fitness (though I hope you've started to see—and feel—how these two modes of training can and should be more similar than dissimilar). At the same time, now that you've created a foundation of fitness that includes endurance, strength, coordination, *and* flexibility, I encourage you to branch out and continue to explore new and different fitness activities that strike your fancy, be they individual endurance races, mud-strewn obstacle races, team sports, dance, martial arts, Olympic weight lifting, or any other type of vigorous movement that seems fun and captures your imagination.

Some of these types of exercise require you to do something I've discouraged up to this point: *specialize*—to turn up the dial on certain aspects of your fitness and, necessarily, turn it down a bit on some others. Now that you're at this level, a certain amount of specialization is actually okay. It's probably even beneficial, as long as you return, eventually, to those areas of fitness you may have neglected. You'll probably return to your old passions with newfound enthusiasm and freshness.

But no matter what you do, always remember the essence of exercise. It's medicine. It's the cheapest and fastest way for anyone to achieve health and happiness. By now, that's something I hope you've learned and will never forget.

May we all exercise for the next 100 years . . . and beyond.

PART 4

The Only Eating Advice You'll Ever Need

I t's ironic. Exercise and eating go hand in hand, flame and fuel, but while there are enough ways to exercise to fill a much thicker book than this one, what you need to know about eating fits in a few pages. It really is that simple—and that important. It isn't about measuring calories or depriving yourself. You're now an *active person*. And an active person needs to eat for fuel and good health. If you eat smart, you'll lose weight, of course. But you'll also feel better and enjoy stronger workouts. Best of all, your body will recover faster from exercise. Smart eating makes exercise a more powerful medicine.

Again: It really is that simple . . . and that important.

The Simple Rules of Smart Eating

"If I were to list the top 10 ways to lose weight," says exercise physiologist and metabolism expert Dr. Christopher Scott, "items 1 through 7 would be why, how, and what you ate. Only the last three would concern exercise." For people who are trying to lose weight, then, this section of the book may be the most critical. But it's equally important for those who just want to improve their health and feel better.

I'm not big on "diet" books. A lot of them don't seem to be about healthy eating anymore; they're more like religious tomes, bent on persuading you that they've found The Truth. The fact is, there are *many* truths when it comes to fad diets. You can lose weight on virtually any diet if you curb enough calories. But few of those diets take into account *exercise*. Exercise requires more food, not less.

It's simple: These are an active person's best habits for intelligent eating. If you adopt them, you'll be properly fueled, feel better, and work out stronger. To help me out, I've called on an invaluable resource—my mom. She knows what she's talking about: Besides helping to instill good eating habits in my brothers and me when we were growing up (thanks, Mom!), Marilyn N. Metzl, PhD, ABPP, is also a psychotherapist and an expert in helping people alter long-term behavior.

It's not easy, she admits, to change your eating habits: "Short of a world crisis—a war or a famine on a large scale, or a heart attack on a personal scale, it can be very difficult to get people to change their habits permanently."

Difficult, she says—but not impossible. The goal, she says, should be to alter your eating and stick to the new behavior for a single month (the same way we do it with exercise). "After that, the new behavior should become integrated into your new way of living."

Here are our simple rules—divided into 2 "sets"—on the best ways to make it happen for you.

SET I: *WHAT* ARE YOU EATING?

1. Get Your Protein Right:

Of the three macronutrients—protein, carbs, and fat—protein may be the most important and the toughest one to get in sufficient quality and quantity. Protein is essential for building and repairing new tissue throughout the body, 24-7. Active people need even more than sedentary folks to replace and rebuild the muscle tissue that gets broken down as a natural consequence of regular exercise—which is why you should try to get *some* protein every time you eat.

For the weight-conscious individual, protein has a couple of distinct advantages. First, it increases satiety—the feeling that you're full and need to stop eating. Increasing satiety, and thus managing your hunger, is one of the more important factors in the success or failure of an eating plan (more on this in a moment). Second, protein requires lots of energy to digest: Roughly one-quarter of the calories that you take in when you eat, say, a plate of poached salmon, are expended on digesting the meal itself. So in effect, a quarter of the calories you ingest from protein are "freebie" calories that won't ever show up somewhere else in your body.

Carbs and fat have gotten a lot of negative attention over the years—to little effect on our collective, ever-ballooning waistline. A better strategy may be to focus on getting *enough* of the macronutrient that (so far, anyway) everyone seems to agree is necessary, good for you, and pretty hard to overconsume. In that sense, protein may actually be the *most* important piece of the weight-loss puzzle.

Good-quality protein is harder to come by than carbohydrates and fat, however, which are available in abundance in convenience stores. Your protein should come from high-quality poultry—I believe in organic, grass-fed, and free-range whenever possible—fish, eggs, and dairy products. Red meat is fine too—just choose leaner cuts (anything with "loin" in the name is a good bet). Whey protein isolate supplements are an acceptable alternative as well.

Vegetable sources of protein, like nuts, seeds, and legumes are not as potent as animal sources—they contain fewer amino acids—but they're a reasonable alternative if you don't eat animal products or there aren't any available.

2. Don't Drink Calories: For the most part, you should limit your intake of liquids to water, tea (especially green tea), black coffee, and, if you tolerate it well, milk. Of these, milk is the only one with calories.

Contrast this with manufactured beverages: Carbonated drinks are the only food directly associated with obesity—the more you drink, the more likely you are to get fat. So if you're trying to lose weight, reducing your consumption of these waistline-killing products should be your number one priority. I include diet sodas in this directive: As much as the marketers try to make you think that stuff is pure and natural, it's mostly chemicals. You don't need it.

Some diet plans, and even some doctors, make the same contention about fruit juice. I agree that apple juice and orange juice aren't the best choices if you're trying to lose weight. They're loaded with sugar (about 20 grams per cup), they're calorie-dense, and most of the fiber from the fruit is missing when you drink the juice alone. But I think most people's diets can withstand a little natural juice now and then. Fresh squeezed is best.

Also: I probably don't need to tell you that drinking tons of alcohol can kill your aspirations for leanness as well. On the other hand, I live in the real world too and think that the occasional wine or cocktail is a reasonable deviation from the "perfect diet" that most people can tolerate. Just keep it down to no more than one a day on average and no more than two on any given day. The only alcoholic beverage I'd say to avoid 100 percent is beer: It's loaded with carbs and empty calories.

3. Easy on the White Stuff:
White bread, rice, pasta, and even potatoes are universally available, calorie-dense, nutrient-deprived foods that most of us eat too much of already. Eating lots of these types of carbohydrates can lower your HDL ("good" cholesterol) and raise your triglyceride readings—both lousy for heart health.

In addition to the worst offenders, I'm wary of most foods that call themselves "whole wheat," too. Most are just as devoid of nutritional value as the whitest of the

DO YOU NEED A WORKOUT SHAKE?

Having a "workout shake"—before or after you put in your half hour to an hour of formal exercise—is a common practice among regular gym-goers. Is it necessary?

The thinking behind the workout shake it this. During and directly after a strength-training session or a tough cardio workout, your body enters a *catabolic* state—muscle and connective tissue are breaking down due to exercise-induced micro-trauma. To reap maximal benefit from your workout, you want to shift into an *anabolic* state as soon as possible, so you can rebuild damaged tissues, making them tougher, stronger, and bigger than they were before you exercised.

That process requires fuel. In fact, you probably need more fuel at that point than perhaps any other point in your day—with the possible exception of when you first get up in the morning. You could sit down to a big, protein-heavy meal in the half hour to an hour following your workout. Or, you could do what the gym junkies do: have a shake.

"Peri-workout nutrition," as the exercise physiologists like to call it, has been a big topic in recent years, and a number of studies have suggested that consuming protein and carbs around the time of your workout can measurably improve the results you get.

Many people wait till after they get home to down their shakes, but it's probably just as important to have a little protein in you *before* your workout: It can take 6 hours for the protein you ingest to show up in your bloodstream, so kick-starting the process before you even set foot in the gym or on the road is probably a good idea. Just don't drink too much or you'll give yourself cramps.

Best strategy? A little in the half hour before you exercise and plenty afterward. If you can get 20 to 30 grams of protein, along with some healthy carbs in your pre- and post-workout shakes combined, your bases will be covered.

white stuff, and some are worse: Stroll down the cereal aisle and you'll see many of the most sugar-laden options legitimately proclaiming themselves "whole wheat" and "high fiber."

Look at it this way: If it's in a package that *tells* you that it's whole wheat and high fiber, you probably shouldn't be eating a lot of it. Stick with super-coarse grains like long-grain wild rice, buckwheat, and quinoa. More great eating: nuts and beans.

4. Load Up on "Real" Fibrous Foods:

"Real" is code for "vegetables, legumes, and whole fruits, and more nutritionally dense foods." Fiber improves digestion and gut health while lowering LDL levels—good news for anyone concerned about cardiovascular health. Notice that I didn't just say eat *fiber:* Again, there's a world of difference between eating whole, nutrient-rich foods that happen to contain lots of fiber, and eating engineered foods with a little fiber thrown in to assuage your guilt for eating it (for more on supplements, see below).

Soluble fiber forms a gel-like substance in the intestines that helps prevent the absorption of certain food-borne toxins. It's found in fruits, vegetables, seeds, brown rice, barley, oats, and oat bran. *Insoluble* fiber, also called roughage, absorbs water in your digestive system and cleans out the whole tract. It's found in whole grains, the outside of seeds, fruit, legumes, and other foods.

5. Eat Fat to Lose It:

This has got to be the most counterintuitive piece of diet advice you've ever heard: Doesn't eating fat just make you fatter? In fact, the right kinds of fat don't. The mono- and polyunsaturated kinds, found in vegetables and plants like walnuts, avocados, walnuts, olive oil, peanut oil, and corn oil, can lower cholesterol, blood pressure, and may decrease your chances of contracting type-2 diabetes. Omega-3 fats, found in fatty fish like salmon, mackerel, black cod, sardines, and herring, reduce inflammation, lower blood pressure, and reduce tryglycerides. In the short term, they seem to help in weight loss efforts as well.

By now you probably know that *trans* fats—of "partially hydrogenated" fame—are deadly, nudging both your good cholesterol and your bad cholesterol in the wrong directions and upping your chances of contracting heart disease. They're so bad that they've been banned in New York City restaurants.

6. Let Supplements Be Supplements:

It's tempting to believe that sports- and performance-engineered food (the ones with the inevitable bionic man graphics on the labels) actually provide something indispensable that you can't get from whole foods. Folks, it's not true: Some of the biggest-selling supplements out there—multivitamins, whey protein, and fish oil—are simply distilled versions of what you get in whole, natural foods anyway. And clinical trials of various supplements like folic acid and vitamin B, initially believed to be heart-protective, have failed to pan out as researchers hoped. With few exceptions, these magical formulas seem to lose their mojo when you consume them in large doses by themselves.

We evolved to consume vitamins, minerals, and vital nutrients in their natural state—as part of whole foods. So far, we haven't figured out a way around that.

SET II: *HOW* ARE YOU EATING?

1. Make It Easy: "As humans," says Dr. Marilyn "Mom" Metzl, "we always favor the path of least resistance." Eating junk food is the definition of easy: It's available everywhere, it's cheap, it tastes good. After you eat it, you get a pleasurable spike in blood sugar and maybe a caffeine jolt as well. When is eating junk food anything *but* easy?

Your strategy, then, is to make good eating *even easier*. Getting the junk out of your house and filling it with the good stuff is step one. Then, learn to make a handful of easy, good-for-you recipes you can whip up in bulk and eat for several meals in a row. If the ingredients are there, but making a meal is too complicated or intimidating in a pinch, you'll just let the veggies rot and call take-out. If a good meal is sitting in the fridge and all it needs is a zap in the microwave and a dash

of pepper, you're much more likely to go for that.

The key to making new eating behavior stick is to know that you *will* get stressed and ravenous at times— and to have a plan to implement when you do.

2. Chow Down Often:

I just ran across a very convincing study, published in 2010, with this title: "Increased meal frequency does not promote greater weight loss in subjects who were prescribed an 8-week equi-energy restricted diet." It showed that, if you control total number of calories consumed, eating six times a day doesn't lead to more weight loss than eating three times a day.

But I'm recommending smaller, more frequent meals anyway. Why? Human nature. In a study, it's easy to control the number of calories someone consumes: Give them a satchel of chow and tell them that's their ration for the day. If they fall off the wagon, they're out of the study.

In real life, it's not so easy. If you're like many working adults, you have a fairly easy time making reasonable food choices through the early afternoon. Then, as the day wears on and work and stress pile up, you don't eat a bite until 8 p.m.—at which point you're so starved that you down the nearest whole pizza, double burger, or mound of pork-fried rice in sight.

It's a common pattern, and it's completely understandable: We all need to eat. The longer you wait to fulfill that primal urge, the more irrational that need becomes.

Again, the key is *hunger management:* You can control the hungry, raging, pizza-devouring beast within by feeding it frequently with good food, so that when mealtime rolls around, you can make the most intelligent, rather than just the most expedient, choice. Studies bear this out: When subjects report eating habits themselves, and the number of calories consumed isn't controlled by researchers, frequent eaters lose more weight, or maintain weight loss more successfully, than less frequent eaters.

3. Stay Mindful: "We're creatures of habit," says Dr. Mom. Once an action works reasonably well, it often becomes a "default" behavior that you repeat, even if there are many better, healthier alternatives available. This is particularly true with eating, which is closely tied to survival: If you had a good experience with Buffalo wings last week, you figure you'll have a good experience again tonight.

The key to changing these behaviors is to drag them out of the murk of the unconscious and shine some light on them. Once you're aware of what you're doing, you can look that choice squarely in the face and decide if you could make a better one. One strategy is never to let yourself get too hungry, which is a major trigger for habitual, unconscious eating. Keeping a food journal, even without

making deliberate changes in what you eat, can also be a very effective weight-loss strategy for precisely this reason: It makes you think about what you're eating. Taking a moment to slow down and enjoy your food before you eat—even saying grace if you're religious—can be a big help too.

As you become more aware of the situations, and emotions, that cause you to overeat, you can take steps to avoid them, or act differently when you encounter them, possibly by eating beforehand or bringing your own food.

Dirty little secret that the diet gurus don't want you to know? *All* of them work more or less equally well, and it's probably for this very reason: Structured diets get you to think about what you eat.

4. Indulge on Purpose: No one is a perfect dieter. The bad-for-you foods are just too ubiquitous—and too tempting—to avoid 100 percent of the time. So instead of going cold turkey on your favorite treats—declaring you'll never eat ice cream, chocolate, or burgers again—*choose* your moments and enjoy them. Buy the good stuff you really like, and, once a week, say, go ahead and splurge, taking your time to savor the meal or dessert or snack. Consciously enjoying your food—even "bad" foods now and then—is part of mindful eating. It's when you mindlessly eat unlimited amounts of junk food, and simultaneously feel guilty about it, that it becomes a problem.

5. Shop the Perimeter: The best stuff for you in the grocery store was recently alive—and goes bad quickly unless it's kept cool (though not frozen): fruits, vegetables, eggs, fish, poultry, meats, and dairy products. The refrigerated areas in grocery stores are always around the store's edges, while the middle sections are jammed with the processed stuff that could survive till the apocalypse. Make it a habit to stick to those outer aisles—with maybe a quick detour down the center aisles to grab some oatmeal, beans, and salsa.

6. Get Specific: We all know the generalities: Eat broccoli, don't eat candy. But few of us *follow* those rules, religiously, year in and year out because we don't have a specific plan for it. Know when and where you're going to buy your food for the week. Schedule time to cook it. Have an action plan for eating at restaurants: a handful of healthy options most restaurants have that don't leave you feeling deprived when your friends are indulging. Generalities fail—specifics work.

7. Keep Your Goals Realistic . . . With airbrushed images of the super-fit, super-lean, and super-ripped on every catalog and street corner, it can be tempting to set your sights on an unrealistic, short-term goal of looking like an athletic superhero in 6 weeks or less. And the diet and exercise books that make outsize claims for instant results don't help matters. Sure—you can go ahead and make getting that super-athletic physique of your dreams a long-term goal if you wish. But in the short term, keep your goals bite-size: a few pounds off a month. Not only will you make better progress, you'll be less likely to throw your metabolism into panic mode and cause you to gain back even more weight if you fall off the diet wagon.

8. . . . But Inspiring: At some point, you've got to up the ante on yourself. This week, all you might be able to manage is cutting out soda 2 days a week. Pull that off and you have to keep raising the bar: How about cutting down sodas to the weekends only for a month? And then cutting them altogether? Put a bunch of those little successes together and the big goal on the horizon will eventually come into focus.

9. Forgive Yourself: "People who succeed in the long run stumble, relapse, and backslide just as often as people who fail in the long term," says the good doctor. The difference is that people who eat intelligently also acknowledge when they overeat—but then quickly get back on the horse and move on. The ones who aren't successful take every lapse as proof of their failure, then throw in the towel.

Perfect, in other words, is the enemy of *successful.*

Acknowledgments

When I first developed the concept of *The Exercise Cure*, I needed to look no further than my sports medicine practice. Every day in my office, I have the amazing fortune to care for athletes of all ages, from 8-year-old gymnasts to 80-year-old marathon runners. Their desire to move and be healthy, combined with my own passion for fitness and health, has allowed me to develop a unique world where healthy activity is the goal. Through these experiences, I have come to realize that exercise isn't only a "feel good" activity, but a powerful and effective medicine that has far-reaching effects. First and foremost, I thank all of my patients, the many thousands of you who have helped make me a better doctor and person. Helping you achieve your goals allows me to learn and, more importantly, to share in your triumphs. I am extremely grateful for your continued support and confidence.

I am deeply appreciative of the Hospital for Special Surgery in New York City for allowing me the space and creative license to develop a medical practice and expertise in the aspects of preventive health that are consistent with my message. My colleagues are among the best physicians I know, and I feel truly blessed to be part of the medical community.

On a personal level, my incredible family of physician parents and brothers has been a continued source of support and guidance for me. I bounce ideas off them regularly, and they are always there to help me fine-tune my thinking and develop new ideas. My family is my backbone. I am so lucky to be a part of them.

Finally, my deep gratitude goes to the family at Rodale Books for believing in this book. Although this makes a powerful case when assembled, taking the risk to make this book was no small step, and I appreciate your faith and confidence in helping me deliver the message. This team includes point men Andrew Heffernan and Mike Zimmerman, as well as Elizabeth Neal and Marilyn Hauptly.

Index

Boldface page references indicate illustrations. Underscored references indicate boxed text

Glute Roll, 116, **116**, 122, **122**, 177, **177**
Goals, setting, 154–55
Goblet Squat, 261, **261**
Gold (advanced) level, 252–79
  determining your readiness for, 163
  month 1, 255–62
    cardio, 262
    strength training, 256–61,
      258–61
    training schedules, 255–56
  month 2, 262–67
    cardio, 263
    strength training, 263–67,
      264–67
    training schedules, 262–63
  month 3, 268–79
    final exam, 269
    strength training, 269–78,
      270–75
    training schedules, 268–69
Groin Roll, 178, **178**
Group classes, 204–5
Gynecologic cancer, 151

H

Hamstring Roll, 116, **116**, 122, **122**, 130,
  130, 177, **177**
HDL (high-density lipoprotein), 34,
  64–65, 66
Health care, money spent on, 5
"Health debt," 7
Health problems
  brain and psychological, 23–45
    addiction, 24–27, 25, 26
    anxiety, 28–29, 29
    attention-deficit hyperactivity
      disorder (ADHD), 30–31
    chronic stress, 36–37, 37, 42
    depression, 14, 18–19, 32–33, 33
    fatigue, 38–39, 39
    low self-esteem, 40–41, 41
    memory loss and cognition
      problems, 34–35, 35
    poor sleep quality, 44–45, 45
    sleep apnea, 43, 43
  cardiopulmonary, 47–57
    asthma, 48–49, 49
    cardiovascular disease, 50–51, 51
    exercising with heart disease,
      54–57
    high blood pressure
      (hypertension), 52–53, 53

hormonal and sexual, 75–93
  erectile dysfunction, 76–77, 77
  low libido, 90–91, 91
  low testosterone, 92–93, 93
  menopause-associated, 78–85, 79,
    80–85
  premenstrual syndrome (PMS),
    86–89, 87, **88–89**
low fitness and, 12–15
metabolic, 59–73
  high cholesterol, 64–67, 67
  low thyroid (hypothyroidism),
    68–69, 69
  metabolic syndrome, 70–71, 71
  type 2 diabetes and
    hyperglycemia, 60–63, 63
  visceral fat (central obesity),
    72–73, 73
musculoskeletal, 95–145
  hip pain, 120–27, 121, **122–27**
  knee pain, 128–35, 129,
    130–35
  ligament sprain, 112–13, 113
  lower-back pain, 114–19, 115,
    116–19
  muscle strain, 104–5, 105
  muscle weakness, 106–9, 107,
    108–9
  neck and shoulder pain, 136–39,
    137, **138–39**, 139
  osteoarthritis, 140–45, 141,
    142–45
  performance plateaus,
    110–11, 111
  poor flexibility, 96–103, 97,
    98–103
Heart disease
  cardiovascular disease, 14–15, 50–51,
    51
  exercising with, 54–57
  heart attack, 8, 10, 11, 14
Heart rate
  for aerobic exercise, 174–75
  checking, 174
  maximum, 55–56
Heart rate monitor, 56
Hematologic cancer, 146, 151
Herniation, disc, 115
High blood pressure (hypertension), 12,
  52–53, 53, 161
High-density lipoprotein (HDL), 34,
  64–65, 66
High-intensity training, 61–62
Hip Bridge, Single-Leg, 134, **134**

Hip Flexor Stretch with Overhead Reach,
  102, **102**
Hip pain, 120–27, 121, **122–27**
Home gym equipment
  chinup bar, 226–27
  foam roller, 227
  jump rope, 226
  kettlebell, 227
  medicine ball, 227
  suspension trainer, 226
Homeostasis, 59
Hormonal and sexual problems, 75–93
  erectile dysfunction, 76–77, 77
  low libido, 90–91, 91
  low testosterone, 92–93, 93
  menopause-associated, 78–85, 79,
    80–85
  premenstrual syndrome (PMS),
    86–89, 87, **88–89**
Hormone imbalances and cognition
  problems, 34
Hormone therapy, 78, 79
Hunger management, 287
Hydration, 55
Hyperactivity. *See* Attention-deficit
  hyperactivity disorder (ADHD)
Hyperglycemia, 60–62, 63
Hyperstress, 36
Hypertension (high blood pressure), 12,
  52–53, 53, 161
Hyperthyroidism, 68
Hypertrophy, muscle fiber, 107
Hypogonadism, 92
Hypostress, 36
Hypothyroidism, 68–69, 69

I

Ice, for muscle strain, 105
IDL (intermediate-density lipoprotein),
  64–65
Iliotibial-Band Roll, 117, **117**, 123, **123**,
  131, **131**, 177, **177**
Inchworm, 99, **99**, 183, **183**, 186, **186**,
  217, **217**
Incline Dumbbell Bench Press, 259, **259**
Indulging, 287
Inflammation
  anti-inflammatory properties of
    exercise, 147
  as memory loss risk factor, 34
Injury
  dynamic rest for, 18–19

TRX Triceps Extension, 248, **248**
Tuck Jump, 82, **82**
Turkish Get-Up, 233, **233**, 258, **258**
Two-On, Two-Off (interval training), 223

U

Upper-Back Roll, 179, **179**
Urine, color of, 55

V

Visceral fat (central obesity), 72–73, <u>73</u>
VLDL (very low-density lipoprotein), 64–65
V-Up, 219, **219**, 233, **233**, 242, **242**, 264, **264**, 266, **266**

W

Walking
    as Bronze level month 1 Workout, 168–69
    as Bronze level month 2 Workout, 174–76
    nonexercise activity thermogenesis (NEAT), 170–73, 201
    pros and cons of activity, 200–201
Walking High Kick, 181, **181**, 184, **184**
Walking High Knees, 98, **98**, 181, **181**, 185, **185**
Walking Lunge, 196, **196**, 235, **235**
Walking Spiderman Stretch, 185, **185**
Wall Calf Stretch, 103, **103**
Wall Slides, 185, **185**
Warmup. *See also* Dynamic stretching
    for asthma sufferers, 49
    sprains associated with improper, 112
Wealth, exercise and, <u>16</u>
Weight loss
    for arthritis, <u>145</u>
    plateaus, 111
    secrets of biggest losers, <u>160</u>
Wide-Stance Plank with Opposite Arm and Leg Lift, 215, **215**, 234, **234**, 242, **242**, 266, **266**

Windmill, Lying Side, 189
Wind-Sprint Fun (interval training), 224
Withdrawal, 24
Workouts
    Bronze level month 2
        dynamic stretching and warmup, 180–87, **180–87**
        foam rolling, 177–79, **177–79**
    Bronze level month 3, 194–99, **195–99**
        body-weight Workout #1, 195–97, **195–97**
        body-weight Workout #2, 198–99, **198–99**
    circuit
        Workout #1, 242–45, **242–45**
        Workout #2, 246–48, **246–48**
    getting the most out of, 154–59
    Gold level month 1
        strength training Workout #1, 258–59, **258–59**
        strength training Workout #2, 260–61, **260–61**
    Gold level month 2
        strength training Workout #1, 264–65, **264–65**
        strength training Workout #2, 266–67, **266–67**
    Gold level month 3
        strength training Workout #1, 270–72, **270–72**
        strength training Workout #2, 273–75, **273–75**
    high-intensity training, 61–62
    for hip pain, 122–27, **122–27**
    hybrid, 210–11
    interval training, 222–25
    for knee pain, 130–35, **130–35**
    logging, 187
    for lower-back pain, 116–19, **116–19**
    for menopause, 80–85, **80–85**
    for muscle weakness, 108–9, **108–9**
    neck-friendly, 138–39, **138–39**
    for osteoarthritis, 142–45, **142–45**
    for PMS, 88–89, **88–89**
    Silver level month 1
        strength workout #1, 214–17, **214–17**

        strength workout #2, 218–21, **218–21**
    Silver level month 2
        Workout A, 230–33, **230–33**
        Workout B, 234–36, **234–36**
        Workout C, 237–39, **237–39**
    Silver level month 3
        Workout #1, 242–45, **242–45**
        Workout #2, 246–48, **246–48**
    for thyroid disease, 69
    varying, <u>254</u>
Workout shake, <u>284</u>
Wrist sprain, 112
Wrist-to-Knee Crunch, 216, **216**

X

X-Band Walk, 135, **135**

Y

Yoga
    for anxiety, 28–29
    for low flexibility, <u>100</u>, 100–101, **100–101**
    poses
        Bow Pose, 88, **88**
        Cat Pose, 88, **88**
        Cobra Pose, 89, **89**, 109, **109**, 197, **197**, 216, **216**
        Corpse Pose, 89, **89**
        Deep Lunge Pose, 100, **100**
        Downward-Facing Dog Pose, 101, **101**
        Fish Pose, 89, **89**
        Forward Bend Pose, 100, **100**, 143, **143**
        Mountain Pose, 100, **100**
        Triangle Pose, 101, **101**
    for premenstrual syndrome (PMS), 87, 88–89, **88–89**
Y Raise, 98, **98**, 138, **138**

Z

Zumba, 204–5